# Global Advances in
# Human Caring Literacy

**Susan M. Lee, PhD, RN, CNP,** is a senior nurse scientist at the Center for Nursing Excellence, Brigham and Women's Hospital, Boston, Massachusetts. Dr. Lee was formerly a Connell Nursing Research Scholar and Nurse Scientist at the Yvonne L. Munn Center for Nursing Research at Massachusetts General Hospital, where she developed and disseminated AgeWISE, a geropalliative educational program, to nurses at 13 Magnet® hospitals in the United States. An expert in the nursing care of frail elders, Dr. Lee is currently practicing what she calls "soul work" as a palliative care nurse practitioner for older adults with advanced dementia and other serious illnesses at the Harvard-affiliated Hebrew SeniorLife. She earned an AS from Labouré College, a BS from Worcester State College, an MS from the University of Massachusetts, Boston, and a PhD from Boston College, where she was awarded the prestigious Dorothy A. Jones Award. Dr. Lee's postdoctoral fellowship with Jean Watson at the Watson Caring Science Institute was devoted to developing a Caring Science–based, mid-range theory called the Geriatric Caring Model. She is delighted to continue collaborating with Dr. Watson on this volume. Dr. Lee, a Hartford Summer Geriatric Scholar, a Hartford Change AGEnt, a Harvard Macy Scholar, and a Caring Science Scholar, has authored over $3 million in nursing workforce grants designed to build nursing capacity in palliative care, evidence-based practice, ethics, and geriatrics. She is committed to helping nurses understand their power to shape the care experience for patients and families through Caring Science.

**Patrick A. Palmieri, DHSc, EdS, MBA, MSN, RN, FACHE, FISQua, FAAN,** is the leading health system and clinical operations expert in Peru. He is a Watson Human Caring Science Scholar focused on shifting the traditional health system paradigm in South America from the mechanical processes of curing patients to the humanized approach of healing by caring for people. Dr. Palmieri is an accomplished leader driven by persons and communities, creating vision, building goodwill, and developing human capabilities, particularly of nurses. Serving across multiple systems and levels, he facilitated change by reshaping the capability of the Peruvian health sector. His work resulted in the first three international hospital and ambulatory accreditations in Peruvian history. Currently, Dr. Palmieri is a professor of health sciences and director of the Institute for Health Sciences Research at Universidad Privada del Norte, Lima, Peru, and a professor in the doctoral program in nursing at Walden University, Minneapolis, Minnesota. In addition, he is an adjunct professor at the Nelda C. Stark College of Nursing, Texas Woman's University, Houston Campus, and at the College of Graduate Health Studies, A. T. Still University, Mesa, Arizona. Dr. Palmieri is an accreditation surveyor for the Accreditation Association for Ambulatory Health Care. He is also a Sigma Theta Tau International Virginia Henderson Fellow and has been named a Fellow of the American Academy of Nursing, a Fellow of the American College of Healthcare Executives, and a Fellow of the International Society for Quality in Health Care.

**Jean Watson, PhD, RN, AHN-BC, FAAN,** is distinguished professor emerita and dean emerita of the School of Nursing at the University of Colorado. She is the founder of the Center for Human Caring in Colorado, a Fellow of the American Academy of Nursing, and a past president of the National League for Nursing. Dr. Watson is a widely published author and recipient of several awards and honors, including an international Kellogg Fellowship in Australia, a Fulbright Research Award in Sweden, and five honorary doctoral degrees, including Honorary International Doctor of Science awards from Goteborg University, Sweden, and Luton University, London. Dr. Watson's caring philosophy is used to guide new models of caring and healing practices in diverse settings worldwide. At the University of Colorado, Dr. Watson holds the title of distinguished professor of nursing, the highest honor accorded its faculty for scholarly work.

# Global Advances in Human Caring Literacy

Susan M. Lee, PhD, RN, CNP
Patrick A. Palmieri, DHSc, EdS, MBA, MSN, RN,
FACHE, FISQua, FAAN
Jean Watson, PhD, RN, AHN-BC, FAAN

**Editors**

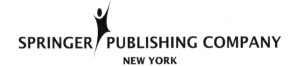

**SPRINGER PUBLISHING COMPANY**
**NEW YORK**

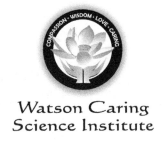

Watson Caring
Science Institute

Springer Publishing Company, LLC
11 West 42nd Street
New York, NY 10036
www.springerpub.com

*Acquisitions Editor*: Margaret Zuccarini
*Senior Production Editor*: Kris Parrish
*Compositor*: Westchester Publishing Services
*Cover Art*: Lou Everett

*ISBN*: 978-0-8261-9212-7
*e-book ISBN*: 978-0-8261-9213-4

16 17 18 19 20 / 5 4 3 2 1

The author and the publisher of this Work have made every effort to use sources believed to be reliable to provide information that is accurate and compatible with the standards generally accepted at the time of publication. Because medical science is continually advancing, our knowledge base continues to expand. Therefore, as new information becomes available, changes in procedures become necessary. We recommend that the reader always consult current research and specific institutional policies before performing any clinical procedure. The author and publisher shall not be liable for any special, consequential, or exemplary damages resulting, in whole or in part, from the readers' use of, or reliance on, the information contained in this book. The publisher has no responsibility for the persistence or accuracy of URLs for external or third-party Internet websites referred to in this publication and does not guarantee that any content on such websites is, or will remain, accurate or appropriate.

**Library of Congress Cataloging-in-Publication Data**

Names: Lee, Susan M., editor. | Palmieri, Patrick, editor. | Watson, Jean, 1940– editor.
Title: Global advances in human caring literacy / Susan M. Lee, Patrick Palmieri, Jean Watson, editors.
Description: New York, NY : Springer Publishing Company, LLC, [2017] | Includes bibliographical references.
Identifiers: LCCN 2016036584 (print) | LCCN 2016036785 (ebook) | ISBN 9780826192127
    (hardcopy : alk. paper) | ISBN 9780826192134 (e-ISBN) | ISBN 9780826192134 (e-book)
Subjects: | MESH: Philosophy, Nursing | Nursing Care—methods | Nursing Theory
Classification: LCC RT84.5 (print) | LCC RT84.5 (ebook) | NLM WY 86 | DDC 610.7301—dc23
LC record available at https://lccn.loc.gov/2016036584

Printed in the United States of America by Gasch Printing.

*To my husband, Bill, and my children, Erica, Christopher,
Stephen, and Holly, who are the greatest joys in my life.*
—Susan M. Lee

*To my wife, Sarita, and my precious daughter, Vanessa, who bring joy and
love to life; to my nurse mom, Carol, for guiding me to join her beloved
profession; and to my friends and colleagues, especially Nataly and Joan, for
helping us advance Caring Science throughout South America.*
—Patrick A. Palmieri

*To all nurses worldwide, who are offering human caring to humanity,
contributing to healing and peace.*
—Jean Watson

# Contents

Contributors     ix
Foreword   Teri Pipe, PhD, RN     xiii
Preface     xv


PART ONE: CARITAS LITERACY

1. Global Advances in Human Caring Literacy     3
   Jean Watson

2. Advancing Caring Literacy in Practice, Education,
   and Health Systems     13
   Susan M. Lee


PART TWO: CARITAS PEDAGOGIES

3. Building Global Caritas Community Through Online Education     23
   Kathleen Sitzman

4. The Caring Science Imperative: A Hallmark in Nursing Education     33
   Jacqueline Whelan

5. The Use of Simulation to Strengthen Humanistic Practice Among Nursing
   Students in the Canton of Vaud (Switzerland)     43
   Philippe Delmas, Otilia Froger, Muriel Harduin, Sandra Gaillard-Desmedt,
   and Coraline Stormacq


PART THREE: CARITAS ENLIGHTENED LEADERSHIP

6. Thinking, Acting, and Leading Through Caring Science Literacy     59
   Sara Horton-Deutsch

7. The Co-Emergence of Caritas Nursing and Professional Nursing Practice
   in Peru     71
   Patrick A. Palmieri

8. Creating Intentionality and Heart-Centered Leadership in the
   Hospital Setting    *89*
   *Jacqueline A. Somerville*

PART FOUR: DIVERSE FORMS OF CARITAS INQUIRY

9. Relational Caring Inquiry: The Added Value of Caring Ontology
   in Nursing Research    *101*
   *Chantal Cara, Louise O'Reilly, and Sylvain Brousseau*

10. Collaborative Action Research and Evaluation: Relational Inquiry for
    Promoting Caring Science Literacy    *115*
    *Marcia Hills and Simon Carroll*

11. Spirituality and Nursing: United States and Ukraine    *131*
    *Gayle L. Casterline*

12. Seeing the Person Through the Patient: A Human Caring Reference Model
    for Health Care and Research    *141*
    *Sandra Vacchi*

PART FIVE: CARITAS PRAXIS

13. Practices of Caring: A South African Perspective    *155*
    *Charlenè Downing*

14. A Conceptual Framework for Midwifery in South Africa    *163*
    *Anna Nolte*

15. Caritas for Society's Safe-Keepers: Upholding Human Dignity
    and Caring    *175*
    *Joseph Giovannoni*

16. Giving Voice Through Caritas Nursing    *187*
    *Maryanne T. Sandberg*

PART SIX: CARITAS PEACE AND HEALING ARTS

17. Caring Practices in an Era of Conflict: Middle East Nurses    *199*
    *Julie Benbenishty and Jordan R. Hannink*

18. Japanese Caritas for Peace and Change    *209*
    *Mayumi Tsutsui, Rina Emoto, and Jean Watson*

19. Caritas Arts for Healing    *217*
    *Mary Rockwood Lane*

*Index*    *227*

# Contributors

**Julie Benbenishty, PhDc, MSN, RN,** Nurse, Hadassah Hebrew University Medical Center, Jerusalem, Israel

**Sylvain Brousseau, PhD, RN,** Assistant Professor, Department of Nursing Science, Université du Québec en Outaouais, Saint-Jérôme, Québec, Canada

**Chantal Cara, PhD, RN,** Full Professor, Faculty of Nursing, Université de Montréal, Montréal, Québec, Canada, and Distinguished Caring Science Scholar, Watson Caring Science Institute, Boulder, Colorado

**Simon Carroll, PhD,** Assistant Teaching Professor, Department of Sociology, University of Victoria, Victoria, British Columbia, Canada

**Gayle L. Casterline, PhD, RN, AHN-BC,** Associate Professor, Hunt School of Nursing, Gardner-Webb University, Boiling Springs, North Carolina

**Philippe Delmas, PhD, RN,** Full Professor, La Source School of Nursing Sciences, University of Applied Sciences Western Switzerland, Lausanne, Switzerland

**Charlenè Downing, PhD, RN, RM, RPN, RNA, RNE, RCN,** Senior Lecturer, Department of Nursing, Faculty of Health Sciences, University of Johannesburg, Johannesburg, South Africa

**Rina Emoto, PhD, RN,** Professor, Japanese Red Cross College of Nursing, Tokyo, Japan

**Otilia Froger, MEd, RN,** Lecturer, La Source School of Nursing Sciences, University of Applied Sciences Western Switzerland, Lausanne, Switzerland

**Sandra Gaillard-Desmedt, MSc, RN,** Associate Dean, La Source School of Nursing Sciences, University of Applied Sciences Western Switzerland, Lausanne, Switzerland

**Joseph Giovannoni, DNP, APRN, PMHCNS-BC,** WCSI Caritas Coach, Watson Caring Science Scholar—Postdoctorate, Watson Caring Science Institute, Boulder, Colorado, and Joseph Giovannoni, Inc., Honolulu, Hawaii

**Jordan R. Hannink, BA,** Hebrew University of Jerusalem, Jerusalem, Israel

**Muriel Harduin, MEd, RN,** Lecturer, La Source School of Nursing Sciences, University of Applied Sciences Western Switzerland, Lausanne, Switzerland

**Marcia Hills, PhD, RN, FAAN,** Professor, School of Nursing, University of Victoria, Victoria, British Columbia, Canada, and Watson Caring Science Distinguished Scholar, Watson Caring Science Institute, Boulder, Colorado

**Sara Horton-Deutsch, PhD, RN, PMHCNS, FAAN, ANEF,** Professor, Watson Caring Science Endowed Chair and Director, Watson Caring Science Center, College of Nursing, University of Colorado, Denver, Colorado

**Mary Rockwood Lane, PhD, RN, FAAN,** Associate Clinical Professor, University of Florida, Gainesville, Florida

**Susan M. Lee, PhD, RN, CNP,** Senior Nurse Scientist and Caring Science Scholar, Brigham and Women's Hospital, Boston, Massachusetts

**Anna Nolte, PhD,** Professor, University of Johannesburg, Johannesburg, South Africa

**Louise O'Reilly, PhD, RN,** Associated Professor, School of Nursing Science, Faculty of Medicine and Health Sciences, Université de Sherbrooke, Québec, Canada

**Patrick A. Palmieri, DHSc, EdS, MBA, MSN, RN, FACHE, FISQua, FAAN,** Core Faculty, Doctoral Program, Walden University, Minneapolis, Minnesota, and Professor and Principal Investigator, Universidad Privada del Norte, Lima, Peru

**Maryanne T. Sandberg, MSN, RN,** Assistant Professor of Nursing, College of Coastal Georgia, Brunswick, Georgia

**Kathleen Sitzman, PhD, RN, CNE, ANEF, FAAN,** Professor, East Carolina University, Greenville, North Carolina

**Jacqueline A. Somerville, PhD, RN, FAAN,** Senior Vice President for Patient Care and Chief Nursing Officer, Brigham and Women's Hospital, Boston, Massachusetts

**Coraline Stormacq, DrPH(c), MPH, RN,** Senior Scientific, School of Nursing Sciences La Source, University of Applied Sciences Western Switzerland, Lausanne, Switzerland

**Mayumi Tsutsui, PhD, RN,** Emeritus Professor, Director of International Collaboration Center, Japanese Red Cross College of Nursing, Tokyo, Japan

**Sandra Vacchi, MSN, RN,** President, Caring in Progress International Association, Turin, Italy

**Jean Watson, PhD, RN, AHN-BC, FAAN,** Founder/Director, Watson Caring Science Institute, Boulder, Colorado, and Distinguished Professor/Dean Emerita, University of Colorado, Denver, Colorado

**Jacqueline Whelan, Academic Associate in Logotherapy, MSc, MA, BNS (Hons.), RNT, RCN, RN,** Assistant Professor of Nursing, Trinity College Dublin, Ireland

# Foreword

*"The life we want is not merely the one we have chosen and made. It is the one we must be choosing and making."*

—Wendell Berry

Choosing to live with intention, awareness, compassion, and mindfulness is an ongoing journey. The decision to live by design rather than by default is a deeply personal one. Yet the decision to grow in this way also has important effects on others as well, especially if we engage in the work of healing and health. In this inspiring book, Drs. Lee, Palmieri, and Watson call upon international Caritas Scholars to expand the ideas of Caring Science to an evolving consciousness of Critical Caritas Literacy. The authors write from their unique perspectives ranging from pedagogy, leadership, inquiry, and praxis, to peace and the healing arts. The writing comes from vulnerable personal and professional growth points, inviting us to share the path in meaningful and inspiring ways. What ensues is a vivid demonstration of the aliveness of Caring Science as a theoretical perspective that actively informs, motivates, coalesces, frames, gives voice to, and amplifies the science and delivery of caring. Caring Science and Caritas Literacy take on the forward-leaning energy of a fluid, evolving, personal-yet-social movement, urging connection with our personal and professional caring core.

This work is an invitation to remember our deep belonging, connecting with self and others in loving kindness with generosity of spirit, rooted in the ethic of human caring. It is this awareness of dynamic self that enables us to more effectively connect with others, be they patients, colleagues, students, or unknown people across the planet. The nature of this work is, first of all, personal, requiring self-awareness and a spirit of disciplined curiosity, willing to *become* even while *becoming* ever more observant and compassionate with the process of *becoming*. The work invites cocreation at every level, from concrete to more abstract, novice to sage, academic to direct care, personal to professional. The work inspires us to reach toward a higher intention for our science, our praxis, and indeed for our very lives, individually and collectively.

The authors engage us to enter or continue in this work with expansive open minds, actively reflecting on how the ideas and experiences shared can be woven into our own lives and work. There is candid acknowledgment of the tension that often exists between the aspirational inner world and the very real demands of care settings in terms of technology, time pressures, and task-orientation. It is in this space and tension that the power of the work can fully come to life. By being aware of and present with the gap between the way things are and the way they might hopefully become, we are more apt to genuinely connect afresh with that which drew us to caring work.

There is a sense in these pages of the ability to enthusiastically begin again and again and again in creatively conscious ways as we take part in a global vision for peace and well-being. There is promise that theory, specifically Caring Science, can and does animate patient-centered care delivery, science, and professional/personal growth. My experience in reading the authors' work is that it made me want to grow-seek-be-learn-become in unabashedly more caring, peaceful, and compassionate directions. May your reading and reflection create even more peace and compassion in your life, and thus in the lives of those you touch and for the planet. For the world needs and deserves peace and compassion now more than ever.

*Teri Pipe, PhD, RN*
ASU Chief Well-Being Officer
Dean and Professor
RWJF Executive Nurse Fellow 2014 Cohort
College of Nursing & Health Innovation
Arizona State University
Phoenix, Arizona

# Preface

This book is a collection of personal/professional narratives from global experts in Caring Science and their journey toward Caring Science and Caritas Literacy. It emerged from a 2015 graduate doctoral retreat/seminar in Lucca, Italy, sponsored by Watson Caring Science Institute (www.watsoncaringscience.org).

Watson's Theory of Human Caring/Caring Science is the foundation for this book. Thus, the original scholarship on Caring Science/Theory of Human Caring/Caritas serves as a guide for this collected work. Caring Science Theory and 10 Caritas Processes have provided a philosophical, ethical, intellectual treatise and blueprint for nursing's evolving disciplinary/professional matrix.

As discussed in the diverse chapters, others interact with the original work in Caring Science Theory at different levels of concreteness or abstractness. The caring theory has been, and is being, used as a guide for educational curricula, clinical practice models, methods for research and inquiry, social–political programs, and humane policies, as well as administrative directions for transforming nursing and health care delivery.

This work posits a value's explicit moral foundation and takes a specific position with respect to the centrality of human caring, "Caritas" and love as an ethic and ontology, as well as a critical scholarly starting point for nursing's existence, broad societal mission, and the basis for further advancement for global caring–healing knowledge and practices. Nevertheless, its use and evolution are dependent on "critical, reflective scholarly practices that must be continuously questioned and critiqued in order to remain dynamic, flexible, and endlessly self-revising and emergent" (Watson, n.d.).

This first series collection of global scholarship in Human Caring Science/Caritas is designed to go beyond Watson's original scholarship and offers a new narrative of "living theory" from the inside out—each author finding his or her own unique way to Caritas Literacy and Caring Science. This collection of diverse perspectives from around the world serves as a historic work for our time, seeking to uncover an evolving consciousness of human caring for nursing and our world as exposed through each author's own personal awakening and from his or her own country and culture.

It is offered as a living exemplar for nursing students, faculty, practitioners, staff, and any and all health professionals who long for insights toward another deep way of purposive being/becoming Caritas in their lives, work, and career trajectories.

The book reveals the global evolving consciousness of each author toward Caritas (love and compassionate service) as a personal journey, transcending differences and uniting in human caring. Each author demonstrates, through his or her personal story, how a worldview of Caring Science and the Theory of Human Caring/Caritas led (and can lead) to new directions for self, system, society, and our world. In some instances, authors depict living exemplars of projects and possibilities that have unfolded in unique ways in their lifeworld. For example, Chapter 17 reveals activities that are guided by caring relations, transcending politics and embedded historic conflicts between Israelis and Palestinians, living caring relations at the grassroots level.

This collected work seen as a whole helps us to grasp how assertive leadership and evolving scholarship in Caring Science, human caring programs, and projects are, ultimately, contributing to world peace.

Finally, this book offers a refreshing dialogue and exposition of Caritas and love of humanity as a forum of living scholarship, demonstrated through experts in the Theory of Human Caring/Caring Science.

*Jean Watson*

## ■ REFERENCE

Watson, J. (n.d.). Theory of Human Caring. Retrieved from http://www.watsoncaringscience.org/images/features/library/THEORY%20OF%20HUMAN%20CARING_Website.pdf

# PART ONE

# *Caritas Literacy*

This book has been written by international nurses who are Caring Scholars. Their stories provide evidence of their commitment to human caring through which they affirm and sustain humanity. In this section, Dr. Watson presents an expanded view of Critical Caritas Literacy, which is an evolving ontology of being/becoming. She contrasts this type of literacy with Caritas Illiteracy, which she describes as task-conscious practices that occur at lower levels of vibrations (i.e., dehumanizing, repressive, controlling, and so on). In the second chapter, Dr. Lee describes her journey to Caring Science and how she continues to evolve Caritas Literacy in her own practice with older adults who have advanced dementia and other late-stage illness. Dr. Lee also coleads Caritas organizational initiatives at Brigham and Women's Hospital, Boston, Massachusetts, a Harvard-affiliated, 793-bed teaching hospital that is a Watson Caring Science Affiliate (see also Chapter 8).

# CHAPTER ONE

# Global Advances in Human Caring Literacy

*Jean Watson*

## CARITAS QUOTE

*While the meaning of literacy is associated with the abilities to read and write, the notion of having fluency in caring at both personal and professional levels introduces a new meaning to deepen our ways of attending to and cultivating how to* Be *deeply human/humane, and how to* Be caring *and have a healing presence.*

*Such literacy includes an evolved and continually evolving emotional heart intelligence, consciousness and intentionality and level of sensitivity and efficacy, followed by a continuing lifelong process and journey of self-growth and self-awareness. This level of evolved Being/Ontological presence is now ethically required for any professional engaged in caring–healing. (Watson, 2008, pp. 23–24)*

*This chapter highlights my expanding views of Caritas and Caritas Literacy as a way of Knowing/Being/Doing/Becoming as humans and as a* universal humanity—*one world/one heart*—*whereby we awaken to the ethical and scientific fact that our being* Caritas for self and others *is affecting the universal consciousness of all of life and planet Earth. It outlines some of the basic dynamics and meaning of Caritas and Caritas Literacy, and evolves* Critical Caritas Literacy *as the ethical and scientific counterpoint to a kind of illiteracy, whereby we witness institutional, professional preoccupation with technological, cognitive, task-conscious competencies, void of our shared human lifeworld—of a shared world of learning, growing, and evolving as caring–loving humans in healing service to our world, sustaining humanity and our survival on planet Earth.*

## ■ OBJECTIVES

*The objectives of this chapter are to:*

- *Expand my personal exploration of literacy—Caritas Literacy*
- *Offer an evolving view of Caring Science and Critical Caritas Literacy*
- *Identify Caritas "Illiteracy"*
- *Provide a personal–professional ethical guide for living and practicing Critical Caritas Literacy*

## ■ JOURNEY TO CARING SCIENCE AND CARITAS LITERACY

Caritas is a journey to the heart of our professional practices and the heart of our humanity. So what do we mean by Caritas Literacy? The term *Caritas*, from Latin, refers to that which is precious and cannot be taken for granted; it conveys charity in the sense of use of self in compassionate service to humankind. In my writings (Watson, 2008, 2012), I use Caritas to depict the deeper ethical–philosophical value foundation of authentic professional human caring practice. Caring Science encompasses all the complexities and vicissitudes of humanity; the term *Caritas* encompasses loving consciousness as the core of human caring, deepening the meaning of professional nurse caring beyond the slogan-like, trite use of the term *caring*, which has become commonplace and even commercialized as a commodity to be bought and sold. Thus, Caritas and Caring Science are grounded and founded on a deep ethical–moral philosophical way of being/becoming more human/humane: a human evolving in higher, deeper consciousness toward connection with the Source—Universal Love.

*Literacy* seemingly is a term known to all. Although it has many meanings, it usually refers to basic cognitive skills of reading, writing, and numeracy (numbers; counting and manipulation). However, ironically in the "history of literacy in English, the word 'literate' meant to be 'familiar with literature' or more generally 'well educated, learned.' Ironically, over time it was reduced to ability to read and write" (United Nations Educational, Scientific and Cultural Organization [UNESCO], 2008, p. 147).

Scholars have debated and critiqued various definitions of literacy and have challenged and expanded the limited meanings of the term. These expansive views are constantly emerging, leading to expanding visions and new questions and understandings of "being literate" and "becoming" perhaps more "literate" at the level of an expanded human consciousness: one who is able to access and process information, knowledge, images, and symbols, and to reflect, critique, and interpret meaning—even construct and create meaning. Being literate extends to the ability to incorporate concrete experience, experiential learning, context, and situations into one's life field. Thus, the term *literacy* has evolved to reflect the fact that there are multiple literacies.

Indeed, as the notions of literacy have expanded, we too may have evolved ways of "being," in which some collective institutional mindsets could be considered "illiterate."

## ■ CRITICAL LITERACY

The vision of multiple literacies has opened the horizon to identify language literacy as an instrument of power and oppression—for example, considering dominant discourses and use of language—that endangers cultures and local knowledge. This postmodern critique of literacy was heavily influenced by Paulo Freire's *Pedagogy of the Oppressed* (2000) and the notion of "critical literacy." His writings and work moved the conversation and use of the terms *literate* and *literacy* beyond the task-conscious conventional meaning of basic reading and writing.

For example, Freire integrated notions of active learning within sociocultural settings. His pedagogical goal was achieved through engaging with books and written texts, but also through reading—that is, interpreting, reflecting on, interrogating, theorizing, investigating, exploring, probing, and questioning—and writing—that is, acting on, and dialogically transforming the world. He also highlighted that the words people use to give meaning to their lives are created and conditioned by the world in which they inhabit.

This critical literacy view can be translated into the lifeworld of nursing and nurses: Nurses live in a subjective inner world motivated by heart-centered human-to-human caring as a moral ideal and ethical philosophical imperative; yet, nurses inhabit an institutional world that is conditioned by a medical–scientific–clinical view of caring literacy as concrete medical tasks and cognitive skills. So "literacy" in the clinical world of nursing is inconsistent with the evolution of "literate" within Freire's worldview; that is, what does it mean to be an evolved literate human being?

The evolution of the concept of "critical literacy" and critique of skill–task literacy is reinforced by the writings of French philosopher Michel Foucault, the popular, postmodern social theorist and literary critic (Foucault, 1980; Rabinow, 1984). Foucault's social–political critique of dominant institutional standards and discourses revealed and reflected how language and discourse control and oppress rather than liberate.

Foucault introduced the whole notion of text and discourse of literacy within the wider sociopolitical practices—for example, we can critique discourse in hospitals by asking the following questions:

- What is the dominant discourse?
- What is the dominant language?
- What is the dominant text?
- What is the power structure?
- How is language constructed to control and dominate health and human behavior? What and who holds the dominant power?
- Whose language controls the discourse?

## ■ CRITICAL CARITAS LITERACY

Critical literacy is close to Caritas Literacy as it has evolved within Caring Science. Indeed, from an ethical and intellectual disciplinary discourse of Caring Science, the term *ontological caring literacy* was posited as a *unitary caring science praxis* to help affirm and sustain humanity, caring, and wholeness in our daily work and the world (Cowling, Smith, & Watson, 2008, p. E41). This evolution of the term *literate* in Caring Science requires understandings of being and becoming as an ontological form of literacy—that is, being literate in ways that relate to critical reflection; the capacity to deepen and critique cultural, ethical, and humane social views and policies; and affecting an understanding of what it means to be human. The "ontologically literate Caritas human," in the way it is used here, is one who is morally informed, with capacity, beyond task-conscious learning and basic survival living toward an evolved heart-centered loving unitary consciousness for purposive learning and living to help affirm and sustain humanity, caring, and wholeness (Cowling et al., 2008, p. E41).

Critical Caritas Literacy asks new questions at the "I-level":

- What does it mean to me to be/become an evolved human?
- How do I practice and sustain caring and compassion toward self and others?
- How can I continue to question and evolve to a higher level of loving, caring, and forgiving consciousness, contributing to caring and healing for self, others, and Mother Earth?
- What informed Caritas acts could I engage in today to be in right relation with others, myself, and my environment?
- What would change if I began each day considering it the last day of my life? Or viewing it as a new beginning—a chance to dwell in humility while surrendering to a higher purpose or guide by trusting in the universe and that which is greater than me?
- What would happen if I dwelled in silence for even 5 minutes?
  - Be quiet for 5 minutes and see what happens.
- Can I simply breathe into this moment, knowing that it is all there is: this moment?
  - All I have are moments. Can I be present to this now, as an *eternal now* . . . just as it is?

• Finally, how do I affirm and sustain my own humanity, caring, and wholeness in my daily work and the world?

Critical Caritas Literacy ultimately is an ontology of being/becoming that comes from within the subjective inner lifeworld of each person, morally aroused for reflective and contemplative self-growth, self-caring experiences that contribute to the whole of humanity.

To better our understanding of Critical Ontological Caritas Literacy, it is perhaps helpful to analyze it against a literary ontology—non-Caritas Literacy: that is, *Caritas Illiteracy*.

## ■ CARITAS ILLITERACY

The counterpoint for Critical Ontological Caritas Literacy, within Caring Science, is *Caritas Illiteracy*—inhumane task-conscious practices; use of lower vibration, objectifying language; "scientizing" of human emotions and expressions; and repressive, insensitive dehumanizing, dividing–separating actions and policies, crafting a commodification of caring and people. Harsh, unkind, controlling cultures within impersonal institutions, corporations, and social networks can be considered illiterate. For example, Caritas Illiteracy discriminates and uses distancing and depersonalizing language—sometimes even abusive, derogatory terms—to reference the "other," who is different. There is evidence of hard-edged words and language that separates, labels, diagnoses, divides, and conquers, inciting fear and distrust as a means of control over others.

This form of Caritas Illiteracy involves ignorance about being human and humane—ignorance about the oneness of the "universal human"; it is Caritas Illiteracy that allows a human to be reduced to the moral status of an object and thus treated as an object, then manipulated and controlled as an object. Caritas Illiteracy is the opposite of Critical Ontological Caritas Literacy, which honors shared humanity through liberating, learning, trusting, and supporting universal humanity—our Mother Earth; one heart/one world.

## ■ GUIDE TO CRITICAL CARITAS LITERACY—ONTOLOGICAL PRACTICES

This section offers a guide to overcome Caritas Illiteracy—the dominant health institutional focus on medicalizing–objectifying humans, as well as preoccupation on technological competencies and industrial corporate measures and practices. Critical Caritas Literacy not only critiques self, system, and society for illiteracy of Caritas, but also poses another way to balance and transcend/transform the otherwise dominant task-conscious literate culture.

## CREATING DISCOURSE AND PRACTICES FOR CRITICAL CARITAS LITERACY

Critical Caritas Literacy involves ontology—that is, a special way of being a loving, caring, compassionate human being, becoming and evolving to be more and more caring, kind, and compassionate with self, others, and all living things. In my 2008 revised book, *Nursing: The Philosophy and Science of Caring*, I developed a section of ontological competencies and Caritas/Caring Literacy as first-level development of the concept of Caritas Literacy. This concept was influenced by others, including Joan Boyce, a doctoral student, and faculty associates in the Watson Caring Science Institute. Caritas Literacy as an ontology brings forth dimensions of the art and artistry of our being; it conveys an evolved and continually evolving health intelligence, consciousness, and intentionality—a level of sensitivity, moral efficacy, and a lifelong journey of self-healing, self-growth, and deliberate spiritual practices (Watson, 2008, pp. 22–23).

## WATSON'S CARITAS LITERACY GUIDE (MODIFIED FROM WATSON, 2003, P. 201; WATSON, 2008, PP. 25–26)

Cultivate personal caring consciousness and intentionality as starting points by:

- Suspending role and status—honor each person's unique diversity—his or her gifts, talents, and contributions—as essential to the whole
- Speaking and listening without judgment—know the difference between discerning and judging
- Working from heart-centered consciousness with others—seek shared meaning and common values
- Listening with compassion and an open heart—do not interrupt
- Learning to be still, to center self while holding a "still point" inside in midst of turmoil
- Welcoming and cultivating silence for reflection, contemplation, and clarity
- Realizing that Caritas transcends ego and connects with others human-to-human, spirit-to-spirit—life and work are divided no more; personal becomes the professional

## PROFESSIONAL CARITAS LITERACY–ONTOLOGICAL PROFESSIONAL COMPETENCIES

The following serve as ontological professional competencies:

1. Sustaining humanistic–altruistic values by practice of loving-kindness, compassion, and equanimity with self/other
2. Being authentically present, enabling faith/hope/belief system; honoring subjective inner, lifeworld of self/other

3. Being sensitive to self and others by cultivating own spiritual practices beyond ego-self to transpersonal presence
4. Developing and sustaining loving, trusting–caring relationships
5. Allowing for expression of positive and negative feelings—authentically listening to another person's story
6. Creatively problem solving–"solution-seeking" through caring process; full use of self and artistry of caring–healing practices via use of all ways of knowing/being/doing/becoming
7. Engaging in transpersonal teaching and learning within the context of caring relationship; staying within other's frame of reference—shift toward coaching model for expanded health/wellness
8. Creating a healing environment at all levels; subtle environment for energetic authentic caring presence
9. Reverentially assisting with basic needs as sacred acts, touching mind–body–spirit of other; sustaining human dignity
10. Opening to spiritual, mystery, unknowns; allowing for miracles (www .watsoncaringscience.org)

## PROFESSIONAL PRACTICES THAT EMERGE FROM CRITICAL CARITAS LITERACY

The following serve as general unfinished ontological guides:

- Pause before entering a patient's room
- Read the energetic field when entering into the life space/field of others
- Maintain the ability to *be authentically present*—be with—versus always doing
- Accurately identify self and address persons by names
- Maintain eye contact as culturally and sensitively appropriate
- Maintain the ability to "energetically ground" self and other as comforting, soothing, calming acts
  - Accurately detect the other's feelings
  - Stay within the other's frame of reference
  - Authentically *listen* to another person's story without interrupting or trying to "fix" anything—knowing this moment of listening is a healing gift for both
  - Hold another with unconditional kindness, dignity, and regard
  - Be able to hold silence with another—create an open space for connecting and reflecting
  - Intentionally use loving touch—this may be noncontact healing touch (HT) and/or physical touch
- Alter the environmental field with energetic consciousness shifts to high vibrational presence

- Translate and carry out conventional nursing skills and tasks into conscious, intentional caring–healing acts
- Translate conventional actions into meaningful caring–healing rituals
- Incorporate healing arts and general and advanced caring–healing modalities and integrative practices into a patient and system care culture
- Discern, critique, and constructively work to change a culture of Caritas Illiteracy into a more enlightened, more open culture and system that radiates Caritas Literacy as the norm

## ■ UN-CONCLUDING THOUGHTS

Simply put, the ontology of Critical Caritas Literacy begins with self, being present and open to compassion, mercy, gentleness, gratitude, loving-kindness, and equanimity toward and with self at the beginning and end. Ontological Caritas Literacy "is a love of humanity and all living things; the immanent, subtle, radiant, shadow and light vicissitudes of experiences along the way—honoring with reverence the mystery, the unknowns, the impermanence and changes that inform and mold us with pain and joy of it all" (Watson, 2008, p. xviii).

The purpose of this book is to help self and others, both authors and readers, to become more literate in the ontology of Critical Caritas Literacy consciousness, moving beyond the task-consciousness, the Caritas Illiteracy of institutions, and the dominant technical practice models.

The Critical Caritas literate nurse and health practitioner become part of a global vision of health and human evolution. Critical Caritas Literacy engages in service to humanity at a different level by radiating the energetic field of Caritas through overt and subtle practices, affecting the whole field. Critical Caritas literate nurses and practitioners become the Caritas field transcending the conventional task literacy by practicing this deep noble caring (Watson, 2008).

In "being Caritas," we become *bodhisattvas* in the Buddhist view; that is, we become those who bless others and become a blessing to self and other. We engage in *unitary caring science praxis* (Cowling et al., 2008). We become evolved, awake and actively affecting the entire universal field of humanity.

## ■ REFERENCES

Cowling, R., Smith, M., & Watson, J. (2008). The power of wholeness, consciousness, and caring: A dialogue on nursing science/art/and healing. *Advances in Nursing Science, 31*, E41–E51.

Foucault, M. (1980). *Knowledge and power.* New York, NY: Pantheon.

Freire, P. (2000). *Pedagogy of the oppressed: 30th anniversary edition.* New York, NY: Bloomsbury Academic.

Rabinow, P. (1984). *The Foucault reader.* New York, NY: Pantheon.

United Nations Educational, Scientific and Cultural Organization. (2008). *Understandings of literacy: Education for all global monitoring report.* Retrieved from http://en.unesco.org/gem-report

Watson, J. (2003). Love and caring: Ethics of face and hand. *Nursing Administrative Quarterly, 27*(3), 197–202.

Watson, J. (2008). *Nursing: The philosophy and science of caring* (Rev. ed.). Boulder, CO: University Press of Colorado.

Watson, J. (2012). *Human caring science*. Sudbury, MA: Jones & Bartlett.

# CHAPTER TWO

# Advancing Caring Literacy in Practice, Education, and Health Systems

*Susan M. Lee*

### CARITAS QUOTE

**Caritas Consciousness** *and relationship call for an authenticity of* **Being and Becoming**—*more fully human and humane, more openhearted, compassionate, sensitive, present, capable, more competent as a human; more able to dwell in silence, to engage in informed moral actions with pain, discomfort, emotional struggles, and suffering without turning away. (Watson, 2008, p. 80)*

*I am a Watson Caring Science Scholar, a title given to those who have completed a postdoctoral fellowship in the Watson Caring Science Institute. Caring Science is the lens of my nursing practice, research, scholarship, and leadership. In this chapter, I describe how I came to Caring Science and its impact on my evolution in this choice and sacred profession of nursing.*

### ■ OBJECTIVES

*The objectives of this chapter are to:*

- *Describe my personal journey to Caritas*

- *Illustrate the intersection of Caring Science and palliative care*

- *Demonstrate current Caritas interventions in practice, education, and systems change*

## ■ JOURNEY TO CARING SCIENCE AND CARITAS LITERACY

Caring Science came to me during the days I sat vigil by my son's hospital bed. Cancer interrupted his life when he was 19, a sophomore in college. The urgency of immediate treatment stole him away from his good friends and college studies to what would be 25 months of treatment for acute lymphoblastic leukemia. During the 3-1/2 weeks of the induction phase of chemotherapy, I sat at his bedside reading and reflecting on the words of Nightingale (1996), Watson (1999), Newman (1999), and Rogers (Madrid, 1997); I was in doctoral study at Boston College at the time with an extraordinary faculty and mentor, Dorothy A. Jones, who was challenging our existing models of nursing, bidding us to expand our vision by considering new paradigms. Little did I know then that Dr. Jones had placed me on the path to Caring Science.

I was thrilled during the times when I did see theory-in-action in the care we received. The very best nurses, unfortunately, were those tutored through their own experiences with cancer. One nurse covered her sparse hair with a turban, an outward sign of the struggle she was living as a fellow member in the community of cancer. She fluidly entered into our lifeworld and addressed our expressed and unexpressed worries from her privileged position of knowing. Another favorite nurse was the mother of a teenage daughter with cancer. She knew what I needed before I even asked—before I even knew what to ask.

During my crash course in oncology, I became a wounded storyteller (Frank, 2013). I felt an enormous responsibility to save my son, to be vigilant, to protect him from the health care system, from nurses who did not "scrub the hub," from student doctors who were practicing on my son, and from the possibility that he would receive the wrong drug or dose or get an infection. I was driven to understand what was next and to prepare myself for what was next and what might go wrong. Being the mother gave me new understanding of the family experience of illness. I chronicled our days in e-mails and my journal to make sense of the shocking diagnosis that our family was experiencing. I journaled so that I would always remember. I opened my heart to the lessons of this illness, for me personally and professionally. As I read my doctoral readings at the bedside, I was puzzled, at times, by the disconnect between what I was reading and the realities of practice. How I wished that the nurses understood the power of presence, not just the physical presence of their being in the room, but the sacred and awesome authentic presence that promotes healing. I marveled that no nurse ever said to my son, "So, how are you doing . . . really? It must be hard to leave college and all your friends to return home for cancer treatment." Those transpersonal caring moments rarely happened for him. On the other side of health care, during my doctoral study and during one of the biggest challenges of my life, Caring Science came to me. And out of those dark hours came my resolution to spend the rest of my career helping nurses understand the power that they hold as healers and comforters through Caritas Literacy.

## ■ BECOMING CARITAS LITERATE

After the first 8 months of my son's 25 months of cancer treatments, I took a per diem staff nurse position in the ICU. I studied and experimented with new ways of knowing, being, doing, and becoming espoused by the Theory of Human Caring. Despite the fact that most of my patients were intubated and sedated, I learned to connect with a gentle touch while whispering in their ears, "My name is Susan. I am your nurse. I know you're very sick but *you are going to get through this.* I will watch over you."

I learned to examine my own biases when dying patients' families could not face the thought of backing down from aggressive, life-sustaining treatments. Their decision to choose life at all costs often caused me as the nurse to inflict suffering, such as suctioning, repositioning the endotracheal tubes, applying tape to faces, obtaining blood gases, inserting indwelling urinary catheters, and so forth. I examined my own feelings about suffering and came to understand that families make the best decisions they can during periods of profound stress and bereavement. Those decisions are often beyond their capacity, given the medical complexity. Their prognostic awareness is not what the team's is, which is likely a protection. I learned to be consciously aware of my feelings and my agenda and to be more generous, more open to mystery and miracles. I helped families to identify miracles that had already come to pass, such as a family member from a faraway place being able to arrive at the bedside in time or a fleeting moment of consciousness.

I encourage all of my colleagues to take risks and try new ways *of being with others.* Fulfillment in nursing is seeing how others respond to a deeper, more authentic presence. In particular, as I have found courage to reveal my spiritual self, patients reveal their spiritual selves; this leads to more transpersonal, caring moments that imprint themselves on the hearts of both the patient/family and the nurse as a deeply human connection. Even in the New England area of the United States, where people are known to be more private about spirituality and faith beliefs, patients/families quite often appreciate being asked about how they are doing spiritually. If you never take a chance, if you never push yourself to try new ways of being with patients, you will miss out on the most marvelous, wondrous aspects of nursing practice—what I call *the magic.* Deeply human connections feed our souls and confirm that we are healers, both in our presence and our Presence. Every connection we make changes us for the better, for the next persons with whom we come into contact. Never before in the history of nursing have nurses been so free in the creative use of self and other modalities in the care of patients/families. We can now, within the scope of RN practice, discuss treatment preferences, goals of care, and what is meaningful to patients. And, then, best of all, we can help to make it happen.

Shortly thereafter, I became involved in palliative care, the care of persons with serious illness. Palliative care emerged as a specialty in the 1990s stemming from the modern hospice movement. Palliative care has its own philosophy of care that focuses on helping persons live with the best quality of life possible while attending to physical, emotional, spiritual, and existential issues. Palliative care, which is interdisciplinary in its approach, was never associated, to my knowledge, with a nursing theory. However, it was striking to me that Caring Science, as an ethical–spiritual–existential philosophy, provided a well-aligned foundation for the specialty for several reasons.

*First, palliative care calls for a qualitatively deeper way of being in relation with others—patients and families, as well as the health care team.* The elements of Caritas Literacy, which Dr. Watson calls "ontological competencies," or people skills, are those commonly used by palliative care practitioners (Watson, 2008, p. 24). They include consciousness, intentionality, centering, authentic presence, reading the field, accurately detecting others' feelings, deep listening to hear behind the words, and so forth. Palliative care nurses often meet persons during the last hours or days of life. Having a high level of Caritas Literacy allows one to quickly form deep, trusting relationships, often within the first hour of meeting. Best practices would encourage the nurse to center first and then enter the room with the conscious intention of being an authentic presence, curious, full of wonder, entering the lifeworld of the patient and family and making sacred space for that which is meaningful to others because the nurse leads the conversation adeptly to the heart of the matter. I enter the lifeworld of the other asking, "Who is this spirit-filled person before me?" (Watson, 2008). In the case of persons who have advanced dementia, I ask, "Who are you *really*? What were you like before this disease robbed you of your personhood? What were your joys? Talents? Ways of being? Help me to bring you in for a few moments so that I can convey a loving presence and a human connection with you."

Caritas Literacy, the topic of this book, describes ontological competencies that are foundational to this deep practice. I wish for all nurses to find their way to Caritas Literacy. I know of no other antidote to caregiver burnout than Caritas Literacy, the processes of which are life-giving, life-sustaining, and joy-filled. The deep, human connection and the knowledge that my caring has been received and appreciated by others fuel my passion for nursing, which has been for me the greatest profession on Earth. And, even when my caring has not been received or reciprocated, I am still sure that the care I gave was the result of my best efforts to connect in a meaningful way. Dr. Watson herself stated that not everyone will receive this type of care (Watson, 2008), but the more I develop my Caritas Literacy, the more I see that it rarely fails to lead to human connectedness.

Palliative care practitioners are often looked to as a healing presence for the health care team, as well, in the midst of intense human suffering, tragedy, and death. The palliative care team is expected to hold an ethic of care, equanimity, and a perspective that will provide calm in situations of uncertainty. Cultivating human caring literacy is important to meet the expectations that others hold for us in this specialty. As a medical specialty, palliative care has developed a lot of training programs in communication. What Caring Science offers is a disciplinary foundation from which nurses can practice in palliative care and hospice.

*Second, palliative care calls for practitioners who are self-aware, self-reflective, and have come to grips with suffering and dying—those who have cultivated their own spiritual practices.* This work is ineffective if one has not lived an examined life. The Caritas Processes are ways of being with others that are deeply and profoundly spiritual. Dr. Watson invites nurses to embark on a new journey to the sacred caring–healing work, "heart-centered connection with our science, ourselves and all others in the universe" (Watson, 2004, p. xii).

Caritas Literacy elevates nurses' work to the highest level of consciousness and reminds us of our moral–ethical–philosophical connection with humanity. Neither the Theory of Human Caring nor the Caritas Processes are prescriptive but inspire nurses to use all ways of knowing, doing, being, and becoming to meet the needs of persons and families.

*Third, palliative care caring–healing occurs within the Caritas field, the milieu that is created with heart-centered intentionality.* In fact, Dr. Watson reminds us that the nurse actually *becomes* the Caritas field for caring and healing, "the magnetic field of attraction for others, offering a new field of compassion and a calming, soothing loving presence in the midst of life threats and despair" (Watson, 2008, p. 197). In the field, the Caritas nurse turns to "things of spirit"—beauty, silence, nature, art, music, stories—as well as material form (Watson, 2008, p. 199).

## ■ MY WORK IN CARING SCIENCE

In this section, I have described some of the ways in which Caring Science influences my work and my being in the world. First and foremost is my practice as a nurse practitioner in geropalliative care. Next, I describe a nursing workforce educational program, AgeWISE, which helps nurses in more than a dozen U.S. hospitals to provide better care for persons with serious and life-threatening illness. Then, I describe my efforts in implementing Caring Science at Brigham and Women's Hospital, a 973-bed hospital that has become a Watson Caring Science Affiliate.

I was fortunate to have the opportunity to study with Dr. Watson as a postdoctoral fellow in the Watson Caring Science Institute. I will forever hold this privilege as the opportunity of a lifetime in my nursing career. To be able to study the theory with Dr. Watson and incorporate it into my practice, education, and research has been transformative. I focused on the intersection of the Theory of Human Caring and palliative care, which shares the same ethical/moral/existential philosophy.

## CARITAS LITERACY: BREAKTHROUGHS TO THE HEARTS OF PERSONS WITH DEMENTIA

The aging demography in America and many other countries brings with it increasing dementia, which is a loss of personhood and memory to those who suffer from this disease. Incurable and terminal, dementia leaves families in its devastating wake with a prolonged period of sadness. My interest in geriatrics came long before my own father died of Alzheimer's disease. Although I had knowledge of this devastating disease, the lived experience was, of course, the most powerful tutor.

At the end of the day, persons with Alzheimer's disease need only two things from professional or family caregivers—love and safety. My prescription for caring is to make sure that persons with dementia receive authentic human caring daily. Long-term care facilities provide activities, games, music, or other activities. I have recently spent time observing group activities and have noted that persons with advanced dementia are more likely to engage and benefit from a concert, for example, if they are positioned within a radius of 10 feet from the performer. If they are outside of that radius, the concert may be perceived as just noise.

In my practice as a geropalliative care nurse practitioner, I spend time breaking through the absent stares to reach the deepest areas of the human soul to deliver loving-kindness and human connection using Caring Literacy—touch, smile, voice, eyes—to convey human love.

Nancy was an 89-year-old widow with advanced dementia who I evaluated to determine why she was occasionally yelling out. I spent about an hour with her one day. At first, she provided one-word answers. Her face was blank. Her eyes were not particularly focused. I asked her yes or no questions, and she answered as she was able. With much prompting, she began speaking in phrases. By the end of our conversation, she was speaking in sentences, albeit slowly. Her eyes came alive. She sat up in her chair and leaned toward me. She maintained eye contact. A nursing assistant who was watching said, "I cannot believe how you were with Nancy. You got her to talk!" Reflecting-in-action, I knew that we had made a deep connection, regardless of the conversation topics. She responded to human presence and loving-kindness from someone who took the time. Over the course of our visit, I told her that she was loved and cherished, that she was a good wife and mother, that her children adored her, and that she had lived a very good life. I told her that she was living in an old folks' home because she was quite old and unable to live alone anymore. She smiled and thanked me for the visit and asked me to come again. Caritas Process #10 is "Opening and attending to spiritual/mysterious and existential unknowns of life-death" (Watson, 2008, p. 31).

## CARITAS LITERACY: TEACHING PRIMARY PALLIATIVE CARE IN AGEWISE

The palliative care needs of persons with serious illness or life-threatening illness, dementias, and frailty cannot be met by palliative care experts; the needs outstrip resources. Therefore, with focused knowledge and skills, all frontline nurses can make a substantial difference for their patients/families. This was the premise of AgeWISE, a geropalliative care nursing education program that was disseminated to 12 U.S. hospitals (Lee et al., 2012). Nurses were educated in communication, ethics, geriatric syndromes, pain and symptom management, and transitions of care. AgeWISE continues to be sustained in a number of U.S. hospitals because it has been a transformative experience for nurses who have been empowered by this education.

## CARITAS LITERACY: A GERIATRIC CARING MODEL

I am continuing to refine a geriatric caring model to guide care to older adults who are in the last 2 to 5 years of life. This work began as an education model in AgeWISE but has since advanced to a mid-range theory that identifies priorities for care and includes interventions and outcomes for frail elders.

## CARITAS LITERACY: EXPANDING CARITAS INTO HEALTH SYSTEMS

Teaching the Caritas Processes among nursing staff in our health system in a variety of ways is another interest of mine. Dr. Somerville's chapter fully describes the overall Caritas plan for Brigham and Women's Hospital, where I am a senior nurse scientist. I am teaching the Caritas Processes to nurse directors in bimonthly seminars. Together, we are conceptualizing a model of Caritas leadership that brings heart-centered intentionality to the lifeworld of nurse directors with the goal of achieving a higher energy field to the entire environment. This work is informed by the findings of a staff nurse survey that identified caring and uncaring behaviors among nurses. The Caring Factor Survey—Caring for Coworkers (Nelson & Watson, 2011)—was used to identify areas of strength as well as needed improvement. Work at the organization and systems levels is needed to build and sustain caring practices for self, coworkers, patients/families, our communities, and our world (Watson, 2008).

## ■ CONCLUSION

The deepening path to Caritas practice, research, education, and health systems change requires an evolving consciousness as well as Caritas Literacy. Caritas is more than generic caring for others. Swanson (1993) calls her theory, which was evolved in Caring Science, the theory of informed caring, which signals the intentionality and knowledge that can lead to creative ways of knowing, being, doing, and becoming. Never before in the history of nursing have nurses been allowed to and encouraged to use their whole selves—talents, personality, knowledge, spirituality, the arts, and conscious intentions—in the care of persons and families. In fact, the mid-range theory of Caritas Processes is ushering in a new age of nursing that is transforming nurses and health systems.

## ■ REFERENCES

Frank, A. (2013). *Wounded storyteller* (2nd ed.). Chicago, IL: University of Chicago Press.

Lee, S., Coakley, E., Blakeney, B., Brandt, L., Rideout, M., & Dahlin, C. (2012). The national Age-WISE pilot. *Journal of Nursing Administration, 42*, 356–360.

Madrid, M. (Ed.). (1997). *Patterns of Rogerian knowing.* New York, NY: National League for Nursing.

Nelson, J., & Watson, J. (2011). *Measuring caring: International research on Caritas as healing.* New York, NY: Springer.

Newman, M. (1999). *Health as expanding consciousness* (2nd ed.). New York, NY: National League for Nursing.

Nightingale, F. (1996). *Notes on nursing: What it is and what it is not.* New York, NY: Dover.

Swanson, C. M. (1993). Nursing as informed caring for the well-being of others. *Image: Journal of Nursing Scholarship, 25*, 352–357.

Watson, J. (1999). *Postmodern nursing and beyond.* London, England: Churchill Livingstone.

Watson, J. (2004). *Caring science as sacred science.* Philadelphia, PA: F.A. Davis.

Watson, J. (2008). *Nursing: The philosophy and science of caring.* Boulder, CO: University Press of Colorado.

# PART TWO

# Caritas Pedagogies

Human Caring Literacy, or ontological competencies, involves mindful, reflective, intentional ways of being that lead to healing and wholeness with patients/families/colleagues/world. In this section, Caring Science Scholars in their formal roles as nursing faculty in the United States, Ireland, and Switzerland inform us of ways of building Human Caring Literacy among nursing students and nurses. Caritas pedagogies are not only relevant to nursing students, but are of great interest to nurses who are evolving a deeper practice that is life-giving and life-receiving. Kathleen Sitzman, a Caritas Scholar, shares the wisdom of Caring Science she has evolved in her practice, research, and education. As a caring innovator, Dr. Sitzman has discovered creative ways of incorporating affective learning strategies through online courses that have reached almost 2,000 people globally, thus expanding global Caritas Literacy. Dr. Jacqueline Whalen of the School of Nursing and Midwifery at Trinity College, Ireland, makes a pressing argument for teaching caring as a moral imperative, as creative art/artistry of all ways of knowing/being/doing/ becoming. Respectful care that maintains human dignity is inherent in relational caring. Dr. Philippe Delmas and colleagues from the prestigious La Source School of Nursing Sciences in Switzerland, who view the teaching of caring as a moral imperative, use simulation to strengthen caring attitudes and behaviors of nursing students.

# CHAPTER THREE

# Building Global Caritas Community Through Online Education

*Kathleen Sitzman*

## CARITAS QUOTE

*. . . ontological shift [beyond modern/postmodern thinking] invites us to recognize the evolving human potential that is emerging from the most recent 20th century [and now 21st century] phenomena whereby there now exists a symbiotic relationship between humankind-technology-nature and the universe. (Watson, 1999, p. 21)*

*Teaching caring through online forums would seem less than ideal. However, as an author, practitioner, faculty member, and innovator, I have found effective ways of incorporating effective learning strategies through online courses that have reached over 1,300 people globally through massive open online courses (MOOCs). My work as a leading Caritas Scholar has enabled me to raise global Caritas consciousness through MOOCs and over 100 printed articles, as well as the two books Dr. Watson and I jointly authored,* Caring Science, Mindful Practice: Implementing Watson's Human Caring Theory *(2014)* and Watson's Caring in the Digital World: A Guide for Caring When Interacting, Teaching, and Learning in Cyberspace *(2017).*

## ■ OBJECTIVES

*The objectives of this chapter are to:*

- *Provide insight through personal narrative into why Caring Science forms the underpinnings of my professional and personal life*
- *Show specific elements of Caring Science that strongly relate to teaching, learning, and interacting in the digital world*
- *Relate how my work in online caring is guided by Caring Science*

## ■ JOURNEY TO CARING SCIENCE AND CARITAS

When I earned a bachelor of science in nursing (BSN) from the University of Utah in 1988, I was excited and optimistic about entering a profession where I could devote my life to caring for others. I had been introduced to Watson's philosophy and science of caring (Watson, 1979) during my undergraduate program of study. It awakened in me a fierce courage and resolve to care and to love, even though overwork, shortages, disillusionment, and burnout were commonplace in nursing. In the first 15 years after graduation, I worked in hospital, home care, and hospice settings, where I encountered a health care system in crisis. It seemed that many people were receiving interventions and treatments with little or no kindness or humanity. Nurses and other health care team members voiced frustration at not having the time or adequate opportunity to truly care for their clients.

Despite this professional climate, I clung to Watson's work as a beacon for what *could* be if we, as nurses, collectively cultivated deep resolve to place caring at the core of our professional lives. Watson's prophetic insights, coupled with her fearlessness at proclaiming the critical importance of deep, multidimensional (and holographic) caring, engendered hope and provided a foundation for what we could build together for ourselves, our clients, our communities, the world, and humankind. I carried Watson's work in my hands (through books and articles) and in my heart/mind/body/soul (through connection at the field of consciousness level) every day. I talked about principles of Watson's Caring Science with colleagues. I wrote over 100 columns and articles for national nursing journals that illustrated the simplicity and power of intentional caring in home health care, hospice, and occupational health nursing.

Many of my colleagues and readers expressed longing to engage in deeply caring nursing practice, but also expressed doubt about the viability of such an approach in such a harsh health care climate. After many years of trying to influence positive change through my own professional practice, I realized that broadscale change was beyond my abilities. I watched many good nurses leave the profession. I became disheartened and considered leaving nursing myself, but in the end, I could not. It was clear that fierce love and caring was (and is) profoundly needed and I felt a responsibility to try and make a difference, however small it might be. Watson's work provided the foundation, inspiration, and guidance for me to assist whatever loving/caring transformation might be possible, wherever I might happen to practice. I refocused my attention on helping individuals and small groups of nurses in varied settings to develop enduring knowledge of how to apply Caring Science at the practice level in the hope of inspiring self-care, peer support, professional resilience, and hope in the future of nursing.

I entered a master of science in nursing (MSN) program at the University of Utah in 1999 so that I could become a nurse educator and teach Caring Science to large numbers of nursing students before they entered the workforce. When I graduated in 2001, I began teaching in the nursing program at Weber State University (WSU) in Utah. The students responded positively to my own Caring Science practice, which involved mindfulness, Watson's 10 Caritas Processes, and cultivating caring–healing consciousness with each client and student. I taught Watson's tenets with simplicity and a great deal of love. Students were very receptive. Regardless of the required nursing content, the students and I always found a way to incorporate an aspect of Caring Science into the learning experience. In this way, I both modeled and taught Caring Science on a daily basis with every individual and in each group setting. I learned a great deal about how to effectively teach Watson's work to students who were just beginning the Caritas journey.

Very early in my career at WSU, I began developing, revising, and teaching online nursing courses. Many felt that it would be impossible to convey, model, and sustain caring in online classroom settings, but I disagreed. Caring and love transcend physical proximity, space, and time. Watson is firm in this belief (Watson, 2002) and I had seen it over and over again in my work with clients through the years, when prayer chains and remissions went hand in hand, when deceased loved ones came to guide a hospice client to a peaceful death, when colleagues called from miles away with a "gut" feeling about a client or situation, and when needed support arrived moments before anyone knew a challenging event was about to occur. I was confident that this same transcendence would enable caring online to be taught, modeled, and *truly felt* by teachers and learners in online and digital settings. Through direct experience, I knew there was great power in connecting with students at the heart level in online classrooms, and I had observed and participated in the conditions under which caring and uncaring occurred in online settings.

With that in mind, I incorporated Caritas language and firm intention to care into every online course I taught and every online communication I engaged in, but there was no research to show the outcomes of this approach. Strong trends in nursing education indicated that online instruction was quickly becoming a standard method of delivering nursing education. I wanted Caring Science to be accepted as a viable foundation for teaching, learning, and interacting online and in the digital world.

I made the decision to earn my PhD, continue to teach, and complete research to clarify the process of conveying and sustaining caring online. I earned my PhD in 2007. My dissertation was on the topic of conveying and sustaining caring in online baccalaureate nursing classrooms. Jean Watson was on my dissertation committee. Her tremendous body of work, coupled with her constant love and support, has given me the courage and resolve to continue my efforts in this area despite many challenges.

To date, I have completed and published eight research studies about the phenomenon of caring online (Hebdon, Clayton, & Sitzman, in press; Leners & Sitzman, 2006; Sitzman, 2010, 2015, 2016a, 2016b; Sitzman, Jensen, & Chan, 2016; Sitzman & Leners, 2006). I have identified simple steps and best practices to support conveying and sustaining caring online. I co-authored a text with Watson that presents Caring Science with simplicity through the lens of Thich Nhat Hanh's mindfulness practices (Sitzman & Watson, 2014), and also co-authored a text with Watson that focuses on application of Watson's Caring Science in the digital world (Sitzman & Watson, 2017). I continue to teach, model, and convey caring online through traditional online nursing education, free and open professional trainings that anyone with access to a computer can complete, and an ongoing international massive open online course (MOOC) entitled "Caring Science, Mindful Practice."

Teaching Watson's Human Caring Science has fueled and defined my professional and personal life for 30 years and it will continue to do so in the future. If my work helps even one person to better understand and subsequently incorporate Watson's work into his or her own daily existence, then my efforts will have been successful.

## ■ KEY ELEMENTS OF CARING SCIENCE AND CARITAS IN RELATION TO CARING IN THE DIGITAL WORLD

Years of study, teaching, and real-world application have clarified for me that every aspect of Watson's work is fully operational in digital settings. Still, I often encounter educators who feel certain that the advent of online instruction is destroying caring as a foundation for nursing education and practice because they are unaware that deeply engaged caring is fully possible in the digital world. The focus of my caring online work is to explore, describe, and disseminate how Caring Science is manifested in the digital world so that others can then envision current and future nursing practice with caring firmly at the core regardless of setting. Key aspects of Watson's work that are important in guiding my ongoing efforts are discussed in the following text.

### LOVE AND CARING ARE PRIMAL FORCES THAT POWER THE UNIVERSE

The following quote forms the basis of my understanding and practice of Watson's work: "Care and love are the most universal, the most tremendous and the most mysterious of cosmic forces: they comprise the primal universal psychic energy" (Watson, 1985/1988, pp. 32–33). It invites us to start at the beginning and then build Caritas practice with the constant awareness that love is the answer to every question—the path that illuminates what to do in times of questioning or doubt. Consistently viewing Watson's work in light of this one quote deepens understanding and enables an intuitive feel for how to cultivate personal caring comportment in self and others.

## TRANSPERSONAL CARING AND THE UNIVERSAL FIELD OF CONSCIOUSNESS

Transpersonal caring relationships, where the one caring reaches out to the heart and soul of the other with love and mindful attention, are central to Caritas practice. Authentic transpersonal caring begins in the moment between the one caring and the individual(s) being cared for, and then moves outward in widening ripples of influence that encompass the broader universal consciousness where limitless healing/growing/learning/comforting/loving possibilities exist. Neither the broader universal consciousness nor the digital world is limited by time, space, or proximity. Conscious awareness of this parity opens a world of potential in terms of engaging in Caritas practice in the digital world. Watson's Caritas Process #10, "Opening and attending to Spiritual/Mysterious and Existential Unknowns of Life–Death" (Watson, 1985/1988), encourages openness and readiness to practice within this mysterious space of knowing and being. In online and digital settings, acknowledgment of the universal field of consciousness coupled with a firm intent to engage in transpersonal caring within this space will allow for unbounded possibilities in terms of teaching, learning, interacting, and experiencing caring in the digital world.

## AUTHENTIC PRESENCE

Many years of mindfulness practice within the tradition of Thich Nhat Hanh have clarified for me that Watson's authentic presence and Thich Nhat Hanh's mindfulness are one and the same. Nhat Hanh describes mindfulness in this way (http://plumvillage.org/mindfulness-practice): "Mindfulness is the energy of being aware and awake to the present moment. It is the continuous practice of touching life deeply in every moment of daily life. To be mindful is to be truly alive, present and at one with those around you and with what you are doing." Watson's authentic presence also requires full attention in the moment, especially when instilling faith and hope: "One of the ways we feel hope is to offer hope to another. Often we discover that in this moment, because we are here [truly *here*] we are the hope; we may become the hope for someone who is isolated, alone, abandoned in the prison of his or her despair and illness, fear and suffering. By being sensitive to our own presence and Caritas Consciousness . . . we may be the one who makes the difference between hope and despair in a given moment" (Watson, 2008, p. 62).

## CREATING A HEALING ENVIRONMENT AT ALL LEVELS

In terms of Watson's work, the definition of *environment* is expansive. It includes visible, invisible, obvious, and subtle dimensions. Personal internal landscapes, immediate surroundings, and the broad external world, to outer space and beyond, are also included. "The interface of technology and human technology changes the basic ontological position of reparation and embraces—or is required to be open to—an ontological position of unity, connectedness, and a transpersonal consciousness and technology that transcend time, space, and physicality. The result is a transpersonal, metaphysical perspective for Caring Science and a new foundational, metaphysical principle for considering the creation of a virtual community of caring" (Watson, 2005, p. 203).

My work is based on the belief that healing environments must be consciously created and tended within all situations, whether face to face or in cyberspace. Healing environments are clearly needed in the event of loss, disease, or illness; however, they are also very much needed in routine day-to-day situations as human beings navigate through an often overwhelming, confusing, or disheartening world.

## ■ HOW I HAVE IMPLEMENTED WATSON'S THEORY IN MY WORK

I have implemented Watson's theory in my work and in my life in many ways. Practicing the Caritas Processes and transpersonal caring moments forms the foundation of my personal life and professional work. Mindfulness practice in the tradition of Thich Nhat Hanh supports deepened understanding and facilitates consistency in my day-to-day Caritas practice.

Establishing a personal foundation in Caritas has inspired a research agenda meant to explore how caring is perceived, expressed, and supported online. The six research studies I have completed thus far have been helpful in clarifying a few key points. Overall *characteristics* of instructors who effectively convey and sustain caring in online classrooms include the skills necessary to write clear/well-organized communications, the ability to sense when students need help, a work ethic that supports promptness, mindful/empathic presence, ongoing engagement with students and course activities, and a high level of accessibility (Sitzman, 2010, 2015, 2016a, 2016b). Specific general *practices* that convey caring online include creating clear and detailed instructions, demonstrating kindness in all communications, sharing of self in ways that let others see the human being behind the text/words/ messages, and demonstrating a high degree of rigor through the creation of excellent work/materials/communications (Sitzman, 2010, 2016a, 2016b; Sitzman & Leners, 2006). All of my study results highlight how authenticity, mindfulness, consideration, kindness, and firm caring intent have the power to transform the field of consciousness in cyberspace (Sitzman & Watson, 2017).

## ■ CARING SCIENCE, MINDFUL PRACTICE TEXT, AND MOOCs

Currently, there is a transcultural/global movement toward informed and rigorous caring in health care and beyond worldwide:

> In this emancipatory clearing for nursing and all health care practitioners, there is another movement towards the making of some common world: a world in which individuals and practice communities transcend traditional professional boundaries and come together to share unabashed love for caring and healing practices, integrating the human-nature-universe relationships in artful, aesthetic, healing practices and bringing together art, science and spirituality to a new depth for those engaged in healing work. (Watson, 1999, p. 19)

MOOCs are administered through universities or organizations that possess the educational infrastructure to host and manage large-scale online courses and trainings. These noncredit courses are offered for free to anyone interested in enrolling. The only requirement is that registrants must have access to the Internet. People who register need not have any formal affiliation with the university or organization offering the MOOC. MOOCs started appearing around 2008 with a dramatic increase of offerings in 2011 when professors from Stanford University (California, United States) released MOOC educational videos and free web resources, and then later established an independent for-profit technology called Coursera to support the creation of MOOCs (Baturay, 2015). The number of MOOCs worldwide surged in 2011 and 2012 and then later decreased as the MOOC concept and technology matured and settled into the broader educational landscape. Today, MOOCs are offered on multiple platforms around the world and address a wide range of subject areas. They continue to provide large open forums for participants to learn about topics of common interest in structured and collaborative learning environments. Dialogue about how MOOCs can best be utilized to provide educational opportunities at local, national, and global levels, while still preserving traditional educational programs/institutions, is ongoing (Brahimi & Sarirete, 2014).

Because the Caring Science community of students, educators, scholars, and professionals includes people with Internet access all over the world, I began to consider the possibility that a Caring Science MOOC could be one way to reach out and provide collective opportunities for connection, inspiration, and continuity—CyberCommunitas—which is an integral component of establishing global caring consciousness. Caring Science MOOCs and other free and open digital endeavors provide opportunities for ongoing connections and exchange of ideas among those who are interested in furthering deep caring in self, others, communities, nations, and the world. Free and open digital gatherings transcend geography, economic limitations, and sociopolitical conditions that would otherwise not allow for the development of significant connections, interactions, and collaborations.

In an effort to create a caring–learning–collaborating space for people to learn about Caring Science, and to openly explore feelings, observations, questions, and experiences in caring, I formed a collaboration that included East Carolina University (North Carolina, United States), Weber State University (Utah, United States), University of Colorado–Denver (Colorado, United States), Watson Caring Science Institute (Colorado, United States), and Canvas/Instructure Learning Management System (Utah, United States), and created a MOOC entitled "Caring Science, Mindful Practice: Implementing Watson's Human Caring Theory." It is offered free of charge to anyone, worldwide, with access to the Internet (canvas.net).

The purpose of the course is to provide tools to facilitate professional caring practices in everyday work environments. Learners are introduced to Watson's human caring theory and then asked to communicate their own experiences related to caring throughout the course. Exploration and learning related to key concepts are supported through the introduction of mindfulness practice, reflective narrative, and contemplative art. Asynchronous discussion, moderated by a team of educators knowledgeable in Caring Science, provides a forum for ongoing interaction and discovery among participants during each 4-week class session. Certificates of completion are earned by participants who complete the entire course of learning modules.

Topical areas include:

- Mindfulness and cultivating understanding of Watson's theory of caring
- Overview of Watson's theory
- Thich Nhat Hanh's five mindfulness trainings
- Transpersonal caring moments
- The 10 Caritas Processes
- Caritas consciousness touchstones for cultivating love

In addition to web links, video lectures, slide presentations, and instructional materials, there is a textbook available to accompany the course:

- Sitzman, K., & Watson, J. (2014). *Caring science, mindful practice: Implementing Watson's human caring theory*. New York, NY: Springer Publishing.

To date, almost 2,000 people from all over the world have registered for the course. Students have come from the United States, Western Europe, the South Pacific, Africa, South Asia, the Middle East, Southeast Asia, and East Asia. The majority of the participants have spoken English; however, non-English speakers have used Google Translate or other free Internet-based translation services to participate effectively within the required discussion boards. Students have had widely varying educational backgrounds ranging from doctoral degrees to high school diplomas and everything in between. In terms of occupational background, nurses and allied health professionals made up the bulk of the students; however, many outside of nursing have also joined. They came from professions as diverse as engineering, retail sales, elementary education, advertising, executive assisting, and many others.

Multiple volunteer Caritas faculty members within this MOOC ensure that students receive continual support and guidance as they work through 4 weeks of

Caring Science content. Student work was insightful and demonstrated commitment to learning and real-world application of Caring Science. The asynchronous discussion board posting areas are supportive, creative, and inclusive spaces where experiences, observations, and insights are shared among faculty and participants. Enduring connections that cross cultures, languages, and geographical distances are often formed among participants. Students continually expressed gratitude for the opportunity to communicate with others about deep caring without censure in an open and nurturing environment. Data from student course evaluations completed after the first offering were overwhelmingly positive, with 95% of the respondents giving the course a rating of five stars (70%) or four stars (25%) out of a possible five stars for overall satisfaction with the learning/collaborative experience. This course will be offered in the future as an ongoing space for Caring Science learning, sharing, and collaborating.

## ■ OTHER CARING SCIENCE WORK: DIGITAL CARING TEXT AND PROFESSIONAL TRAININGS

I collaborated with Jean Watson to write a handbook about conveying and sustaining caring in cyberspace, *Watson's Caring in the Digital World: A Guide for Caring When Interacting, Teaching, and Learning in Cyberspace* (Sitzman & Watson, 2017). The topical areas include viewing Watson's theory within the context of cyberspace, utilizing CyberCaring in online classrooms, expressing caring in cyberspace communications, and expressing global intent to care through offering a Caring Science, Mindful Practice MOOC. This handbook is an easy reference for simple evidence-based practices that will support caring in cyberspace.

I also wanted to provide independent study options for people who want to learn more about caring. I created two free and open trainings that are offered on my institution's website for anyone who has access to the Internet:

- Conveying and Sustaining Caring in Online Classrooms
- Mindful Communication for Caring Online

These trainings are convenient for people who need to learn independently at their own pace during any time period that is convenient for them. To date, 80 people locally, nationally, and internationally have completed training. Both trainings will be offered in the future, with plans of adding additional trainings as time allows.

## ■ CONCLUSION

As my work unfolds under the lens of human caring theory, I am constantly reminded that miracles will enter if welcomed. I have learned through many years of working with Jean and with Caring Science that the willingness to open my heart to loving-kindness and mystery ushers in serendipity, opportunity, and extraordinary connection. I see love, or the potential for love, everywhere.

> In my mind
> The question is not
> "Is love possible?"
> It is always
> "How can I coax it into the light?"

—*K. Sitzman*

## ■ REFERENCES

Baturay, M. H. (2015). An overview of the world of MOOCs. *Procedia-Social and Behavioral Sciences, 174*, 427–433.

Brahimi, T., & Sarirete, A. (2014). Learning outside the classroom through MOOCs. *Computers in Human Behavior, 51*, 604–609.

Hebdon, M., Clayton, M., & Sitzman, K. (2016). Caring intention transformation in an interprofessional massive open online course. *International Journal for Human Caring, 20*(4), in press.

Leners, D. W., & Sitzman, K. (2006). Graduate student perceptions: Feeling the passion of caring online. *Nursing Education Perspectives, 27*(6), 315–319.

Sitzman, K. (2010). Student-preferred caring behaviors for online nursing education. *Nursing Education Perspectives, 31*(3), 171–178.

Sitzman, K. (2015). Sense, connect, facilitate: Nurse educator experiences of caring through Watson's lens. *International Journal for Human Caring, 19*(3), 25–29.

Sitzman, K. (2016a). Mindful communication for caring online. *Advances in Nursing Science, 39*(2), 37–46.

Sitzman, K. (2016b). What student cues prompt online instructors to offer caring interventions? *Nursing Education Perspectives, 37*(2), 61–71.

Sitzman, K., Jensen, A., & Chan, S. (2016). Creating a global community of learners in nursing and beyond: Caring science, mindful practice massive open online course. *Nursing Education Perspectives, 37*(5), 269–274.

Sitzman, K., & Leners, D. (2006). Student perceptions of caring in online baccalaureate education. *Nursing Education Perspectives, 27*(5), 254–259.

Sitzman, K., & Watson, J. (2014). *Caring science, mindful practice: Implementing Watson's human caring theory.* New York, NY: Springer Publishing.

Sitzman, K., & Watson, J. (2017). *Watson's caring in the digital world: A guide for caring when interacting, teaching, and learning in cyberspace.* New York, NY: Springer Publishing.

Watson, J. (1979). *The philosophy and science of caring.* Boston, MA: Little Brown.

Watson, J. (1985/1988). *Nursing: Human science and human care.* New York, NY: National League for Nursing.

Watson, J. (1999). *Postmodern nursing and beyond.* London, England: Churchill Livingstone.

Watson, J. (2002). Metaphysics of virtual caring communities. *International Journal for Human Caring, 6*(1), 41–45.

Watson, J. (2005). *Caring science as sacred science.* Philadelphia, PA: F.A. Davis.

Watson, J. (2008). *Nursing: The philosophy and science of caring* (Rev. ed.). Boulder, CO: University Press of Colorado.

CHAPTER FOUR

# The Caring Science Imperative: A Hallmark in Nursing Education

Jacqueline Whelan

## CARITAS QUOTE

*Human caring can be most effectively demonstrated and practiced only interpersonally. The intersubjective human process keeps alive a common sense of humanity; it teaches us how to be human by identifying ourselves with others, whereby the humanity of one is reflected in the other. (Watson, 2012, pp. 43–44)*

*This chapter maps my personal journey to Caring Science, philosophical worldview, and educational influences in nursing, education, and beyond. It considers challenges in addressing caring as a domain of nursing. The contribution of Dr. Watson's theory is considered. The current position of caring in nursing in Ireland is provided.*

## ◼ OBJECTIVES

*The objectives of this chapter are to:*

- *Describe my personal journey to Caring Science*
- *Illustrate ways of knowing/being/doing/becoming in Caring Science*
- *Demonstrate the need for caring theory-guided pedagogies*

## ■ JOURNEY TO CARING SCIENCE AND CARITAS LITERACY

My introduction to Caring Science began in 1994. It started with a philosophy class in the Faculty of Medicine at University College Dublin (UCD), the only university in the Republic of Ireland that provided a third-level education for prospective nurse educators. Sr. Triona Harvey, a lecturer in the Department of Nursing Studies, raised the subject of caring and its relationship to nursing. Given nursing's professional mandate to care, it was stressed that nursing needs to justify and legitimize its need to care through making caring visible rather than invisible. Reference was made to Leininger and Watson's (1990) book, *The Caring Imperative in Education*, which resonated with me as a means of instilling new ways of knowing in nursing. I remember pausing, reflecting, and experiencing a distinct point of clarity, a light bulb moment. I was intrigued. This moment culminated in the realization of nursing's raison d'être through care, constituting an inherent life force. I recognized that caring was the fundamental core value that mattered most in order to address both nursing and societal concerns, perceptions, meanings, needs, and expectations as a means of transforming the health care landscape.

Although caring was universally accepted as an inherent core value, through my professional experience I became increasingly aware that caring was elusive, invisible, largely unexplored, and very loosely applied in the context of nursing and nursing education in the early 1990s in my country. Space was not created in behaviorally based, content-led curricula systems that existed at that time to examine the pivotal role of caring in the discipline of nursing; in contrast, the National League for Nursing (NLN) in the United States developed a curriculum revolution culminating in the development of caring as a core nursing curricular value (Tanner, 1990). The question for me was why caring was not treated respectfully as a distinct core value in nursing; why was it not placed center stage at the very heart of nursing education and practice? This new perspective drew me in as caring linguistics, caring principles, and caring practices were not ordinarily articulated, acknowledged, or understood as a norm within nursing.

On reflection, my worldview has always been oriented toward a philosophical, epistemological lens that concerns what matters most: humanity, existence, being, meaning, and purpose. I was immediately drawn to Dr. Watson's theory given its inherent tridimensional approach—art, science, and humanities—that posited a theory of human conscious caring in order to develop a more meaningful transcendental approach to nursing through relatedness and relationship-centered care. This demanded an extended view of nursing's conventional metaparadigm that considers caring as a moral ideal and acknowledges the spiritual dimension and metaphysical aspects of nursing (Watson, 1988). This unique philosophical holistic view regarded caring as the highest ethical ideal, the intentionality of our humanity coupled with the notion of alignment to come into right relation, to help others find meaning in suffering and death, to preserve and deepen humanity, and to sustain caring, particularly where it is threatened. The philosophical underpinnings of the theory spoke to the expansive ontological perspective of belonging, being, and becoming. Informed by the work of Levinas, "ethics of face," sustaining humanity through spirit-to-spirit connection between a nurse and a patient was revolutionary (Watson, 2005). This, in essence, is what nursing is all about for me: a sacred privileged journey, prioritizing and placing a value on maintaining interpersonal aspects of relatedness, purposeful holding, and touching the life force and humanity of another person in order to help that person heal, recover, or have a peaceful death.

The notion of ontological development was very new to me. Both Roach's (1984) and Benner and Wrubel's (1989) work further informed my thinking. This made me more mindful, more present, more intentional, with the aim of transforming my thinking, myself, and my students with a view to attempting to change the educational field.

Watson's initial primary value system and carative factors represented a tentative framework in actually classifying the body of nursing knowledge for the study and practice of caring (Boykin, 1994). It provided a path for emphasizing a humanistic and scientific direction wholly commensurate with nursing practice aims (Cohen, 1991). Furthermore, the factors acted as cues for students to relay attitudes and intentions that emanate from the nurse–patient relationship (Boykin, 1994). Fundamentally, it sought to redress the core of nursing (nurse–patient relationship) as distinct from the "trim" of nursing captured by tasks, procedures, and techniques. The subsequent refinement of the theory with the development of Caritas Processes propelled the Caring Science Theory forward, culminating in core principles, concepts, and practices akin to nursing's aims.

The pursuit of subsequent study led me to *An Exploratory Study of the Meaning and Experience of Caring; Staff Nurses Perspectives* (Whelan, 1995) in order to make sense of how caring is created and understood in the nursing world. This particular interest was further advanced through undertaking a master of science in nursing (Royal College of Nursing London)—*The Caring Dimension in Nursing Education: A Hermeneutic Enquiry of Students' Perspectives of the Meaning and Experience of Caring* (Whelan, 2003). I was driven to undertake the *International Certificate Program in Caring and Healing* led by Dr. Jean Watson in May 2007 and her wonderful faculty—Drs. Sally Gadow, Janet Quinn, and Cynthia Hutchinson—at the University of Colorado. This cultivated a deep interest in coalescing spirituality with caring as a developmental process. To feed my philosophical interests further, I commenced an Academic Associate program of study in logotherapy, "meaning centered therapy," with the Viktor Frankl Institute in Dublin in 2013 under the direction of Dr. Stephen Costello. This program has been transformative in helping me to understand Frankl's perspective in asserting existential freedom and responsibility as the grounds for spiritual being and actualizing meaning in life (Frankl, 1992). Another progressive development, *The Spirituality Interest Group* (an umbrella interest group developed in the School of Nursing and Midwifery in Trinity College Dublin set up by Dr. Timmins), represents a creative interdisciplinary international research space to increase awareness, discussion, and debate toward an integral understanding of the need and associated roles to provide spiritual care in health care (Timmins, Murphy, Caldeira, et al., 2016; Timmins, Murphy, Pujol, et al., 2016).

Contextually, a recent research survey regarding public attitudes toward Irish nurses and midwives found them to have high ethical standards and high caring and compassion ratings in patient care (Amarach, 2013). However, this position is juxtaposed against other notable reports that have tested the profession's understanding of the professional concept of care and the value of caring (Harding Clark, 2006; Health Information Quality Authority [HIQA], 2013, 2015; Health Service Executive, 2006). A recent values-based initiative was undertaken by the Chief Nursing Officer, Department of Health, in partnership with the Office of Nursing and Midwifery Services Director (ONMSD) HSE, and the President of the Nursing and Midwifery Board of Ireland (NMBI; O'Halloran, Wynne, & Cassidy, 2016). Nurses and midwives were asked to identify and develop a relational set of values and to consider behaviors and skills that could be implemented in practice. This initiative culminated in an extensive national consultation process and development of a position paper that identified and agreed on Compassion, Care, and Commitment as the three distinct core values that underpin nursing and midwifery practice in Ireland. It is wonderful to witness the profession coming full circle by recognizing, valuing, supporting, and sustaining these values as guiding principles of nursing education, practice, and management. Ultimately for me, being in the world is contained and realized in being, in care, and through caring. This perspective and energy is fundamental to my understanding of life and work as it is currently constructed.

## ■ ALL WAYS OF KNOWING/BEING/DOING/BECOMING

Caring in nursing represents the most substantive concept that nurse educators have to work with, as caring values, caring attitudes, and caring behaviors represent distinct components of the professional nurse education process. For Dr. Watson, caring is the essence of nursing. It is a fundamental requirement and constitutes a professional responsibility, rooted in ethical concern and commitment required for purposeful engagement to nurture and protect the welfare of humanity. As a nurse educator, I am challenged to comprehend how students may come to know caring, how it may be nurtured to create meaning and socialized as a distinct core value to help students develop human caring abilities and responses. As such, this has implications for how caring is communicated, modeled, and learned in education and practice, as students move from personal to professional aspects of communicating caring. This raises the question of how educators can best prepare students to develop professional caring knowledge, caring attitudes, behaviors, actions, and competent skills commensurate with safe effective patient care and outcomes in practice.

The process of nurse education demands that we question the very nature of Caring Science knowledge, teaching, and learning of Caring Science, which simply cannot be inferred or mean that individuals will practice caring (Roach, 1984;

Watson & Smith, 2002). Students may choose nursing as a career out of a desired commitment to care; however, a dormant response may exist and persist if caring is not acknowledged or nurtured (Roach, 1984). A caring response may be increased or suppressed in a student given the nature of the educational experience to which students are subjected. Research has concluded that caring must be role modeled by faculty for students to practice caring (Gramling & Nugent, 1998). Moreover, it has been demonstrated that students' personal qualities may not alter as a result of the educational process (Gramling & Nugent, 1998). Research has also asserted that graduates experience problems maintaining value sets obtained during their educational program due to environmental factors, which mitigate an additional theory–practice divide (Maben, Latter, & Clark, 2007; Pitt, Powis, Levett-Jones, & Hunter, 2014). What these studies clearly demonstrate is that caring experiences may not be universal in nursing students and that caring cannot be merely *caught* over the course of a program. Rather, what is required is for caring to be clearly structured and embedded within undergraduate and postgraduate curricula, and beyond. In spite of varying debates in the literature regarding whether caring can be taught, or considered to be a process, nursing has been criticized for not adequately considering the process of education required in the preparation of nurses as all-encompassing caring individuals. It follows that students be orientated toward ethical values-based education where distinct core values of the nursing profession are taught, justified, and understood (Arnold & Underman Boggs, 2015). Caring outcomes are dependent on teaching caring in order to sensitize students to all professional caring aspects aligned to professional practice.

Thus, caring conceptually requires an expansive lens, multiple ways of knowing, that Dr. Watson's theory fulfills as essential tools for instigating human caring practices as a means of understanding, finding meaning, and transformation in professional nursing practice (Bonis, 2009; Rycroft-Malone et al., 2004). This expanded view requires an integrative teaching approach for the purposes of teaching communication caring theory and skills and an interpersonal process to promote opportunities for teacher–student engagement in order to nurture Caring Science as the ethical ideal in nursing (MacDonald-Wicks & Levett-Jones, 2012).

An essential function of theory in nursing education rests with directing nursing practice and is not merely theory for the sake of addressing theoretical concerns. Dr. Watson's Caring Science Theory represents a consolidated heart-filled centered practice, as it combines caring (a euphemism for loving) that demonstrates the need for conscious supportive interventions through 10 Caritas Processes. It converges a pluralist type of knowing by addressing philosophical, empirical, ethical, personal, and aesthetic forms of knowing (from nursing and other disciplines), all seminal to the student nurses getting to know and understand themselves in relation to the world they live in as people first. Located within a transpersonal perspective that allows generation of meaning and feelings, Dr. Watson's theory cultivates how we come to be in relation to others through the creation of conscious awareness and understandings of the need for care, and cultural and spiritual awareness as core understandings (Carper, 1978; Watson, 2005, 2008).

Dr. Watson's philosophical foundations of belonging, being, and doing of Caring Science and its convergence with unitary science hold relevance for how we should view humanity and engagement when caring for others. Dr. Watson's (Levinas, cited by Watson 2005, p. 44) key philosophical element of "ethics of face" is seminal as it reminds us that we need to open ourselves to humanity, instead of closing ourselves off to inhumane care practices. It demands us to confront the face of humanity, like a mirror glass, in order to consider what is seen, reflected back, and what is mirrored through person-to-person interactions. This constitutes a deep-seated connection when encountering the face of another person. Taking account of Levinas' element when caring, it is postulated that we are literally holding sacred space for the mystery of life of another in our hands that cannot be abandoned and alienated (Watson, 2005). This reverential encountering position represents a reality, a truth that articulates a sense of oneness in that we all belong to one another before we come to be (Watson, 2005). This position allows us to confront and uphold the life force of another instead of adopting a separatist perspective that exemplifies a mind–body–spirit split (Watson, 2005).

Watson's use of a second philosophical key element, "ethical demand" (Logstrup, cited by Watson, 2005, p. 51), proposes that reality is perceived through holding the life of another person in our hands. This view emerges not from an individualistic viewpoint but rather from a position of vulnerability. Ethical demand requires us to forget ourselves in order to dedicate ourselves to a higher cause. By enmeshing ourselves in the life of another, this reinforces our sense of humanity. Life is not constructed by us; rather, it is construed as a reciprocal interpersonal process as a condition of our existence (engaged in giving and receiving) underpinned by a sense of care, trust, and selfless expressions.

The relational holistic dimensions of Watson's theory acknowledge a spiritual domain that draws on spiritual existential knowing as an aspect of Caring Science; this relates to helping patients find meaning and meaning making in the face of adversity and finding purpose in patient lives. This raises the question as to how nurses can come to know a patient's spiritual reality when confronted with illness, suffering, death, and adversity (Watson, 2005). How can we assist students to "encounter sickness until death" (Watson, 2005, p. xi)? How can we instill hope in the life of a patient who may be vulnerable, resulting in an existential crisis and spiritual distress? Individuals have a right to have their spiritual needs met whether they believe in having a soul or not. Watson contends that it is precisely the nurse caring and the transactions that unfold which contribute to the patient's understanding of his or her beliefs and purpose in life as a distinct concern (Watson, 2005).

From a Caring Science perspective, it means that we need to turn the student's attention to many gifts and dimensions associated with transpersonal unitary caring theory, to become conscious of the responsibility that a student holds toward confronting humanity of self, of the other (patient) through caring (Watson, 2005). Through these philosophies, Dr. Watson captures our authentic sense of belonging and connectedness in order to orientate ourselves toward responsibility (Watson, 2005). Both key philosophical elements aspire to the affinity of belonging that allows us to create space to come to know and understand how we come to be orientated (individual, societal, and global levels); to consider what is good and right; and identify what serves individuals' and patients' best interests. These perspectives comprehend essentially how humanity and the *self* are all universally connected and orientated through relational encounters that connect belonging and being, and thus becoming infinite.

The development of the student nurse educator and student nurse–patient relationship is crucial in order to take responsibility for and best place the student and patient at the center of all educational and practice care interventions. This means that students' capacity for learning relational caring communication must be realized and nurtured in education as an important entity in the covert and overt aspects of the curriculum for students in order to prevent a dormant caring response (Roach, 1984). Relational caring of Watson's theory is underpinned by the distinct professional values of respect and dignity as quality expectations for the person across the life span aligned to the first Caritas Process. Given that patients may not be treated with a deserved sense of respect or dignity maintenance (Baillie & Gallagher, 2009), educators need to consider how they model and convey respect in the educational environment with a view to understanding how students demonstrate mutual respect for self and others (Clucas & Chapman, 2014). Respectful care needs to be all encompassing and adopt a broad scope that embraces kindness and sensitivity underpinned by frameworks that promote the development of compassion and embrace a relational cultural lens framework for students to become culturally competent.

Students need to be given an opportunity to consider how they should promote, protect, and maintain the patient's dignity through particular care activities in addition to understanding students', patients', and nurses' perceptions of dignity and those activities that may potentially compromise dignity in practice (Royal College of Nursing, 2008). This is in keeping with Watson's view of human dignity preservation that sustains what Frankl calls his tridimensional ontology, unification of mind, body, and spirit.

Taking responsibility and accountability in caring for a patient's life can either promote growth and sustain a patient's illness or well-being or stifle a patient's life. Students need to be given opportunities to clarify and dialogue their caring values, care for self, caring acts of kindness, caring moments, caring processes, and caring outcomes they have experienced as ways of knowing caring with a view to sensitizing and guiding students' moral, ethical, and personal development of caring. This allows students to pay attention, to listen, to engage in meaningful caring as distinct from viewing caring as a mere ritualistic event and to further draw on distinctions between caring and noncaring encounters with patients. If students witness or experience noncaring in either nursing education and/or practice, students may be socialized to accept this practice as a norm, which mitigates against embracing a

Caring Science perspective. Values clarification exercises and techniques extended beyond undergraduate programs of study to postgraduate level are beneficial in assisting students to test, break down, and clarify previously held values. This asserts a student's thinking and behavior, thus questioning the student's responsibility and accountability for his or her ethical choices and determinations when caring.

## ■ CONCLUSION

My path to Caritas has been evolving for many years and is consistent with my worldview that has always been oriented toward caring, humanity, existence, being, meaning, and purpose. From an educator's perspective, helping students develop caring literacy is a moral imperative because caring is the very essence of nursing. How we, as educators, instill and nurture caring among students is vital—through respect for humanity, dignity, and body/mind/spirit holism. Students are not in a position to assist patients until they have clarity around their concepts of self, self-care, behavior, feelings, and actions, which requires multiple ways of knowing and understanding as an aspect of nurse–patient relationships (Wagner & Seymour, 2007). This requires expert caring guidance along with practice, reflection, and dialogue—all ways of knowing/being/doing/becoming.

## ■ REFERENCES

Amarach. (2013). *Public attitudes to nurses and midwives.* An Amarach Research Survey for An Bord Altranais (Nursing Board), Dublin. Retrieved from www.slideshare.net/amarach/irish-attitudes -to-nurses-and-midwives

Arnold, E. C., & Underman Boggs, K. (2015). *Interpersonal relationships: Professional communication skills for nurses* (7th ed.). St. Louis, MO: Saunders.

Baillie, L., & Gallagher, A. (2009). Evaluation of the Royal College of Nursing's "Dignity: At the Heart of Everything We Do" campaign: Exploring challenges and enablers. *Journal of Research in Nursing, 15,* 15–28. Retrieved from http://jrn.sagepub.com/content/15/1/15.full.pdf+html

Benner, P., & Wrubel, J. (1989). *The primacy of caring: Stress and coping in health and illness.* Menlo Park, CA: Addison-Wesley.

Bonis, S. A. (2009). Knowing in nursing: A concept analysis. *Journal of Advanced Nursing, 65,* 1328–1341. Retrieved from www.ncbi.nlm.nih.gov/pubmed/19291190

Boykin, A. (1994). Creating a caring environment for nursing education. In A. Boykin (Ed.), *Living a caring based program* (pp. 11–25). New York, NY: National League for Nursing.

Carper, B. (1978). Fundamental patterns of knowing. *Advances in Nursing Science, 1,* 13–23. Retrieved from journals.lww.com/advancesinnursingscience/Citation/1978/10000/Fundamental_Patterns_of _Knowing_in_Nursing_.4.aspx

Clucas, C., & Chapman, H. M. (2014). Respect in final-year student nurse–patient encounters: An interpretative phenomenological analysis. *Health Psychology & Behavioral Medicine, 2,* 671–685.

Cohen, J. (1991). Two portraits of caring: A comparison of artists, Leininger and Watson. *Journal of Advanced Nursing, 16,* 899–909. Retrieved from www.ncbi.nlm.nih.gov/pubmed/1779078

Frankl, V. (1992). *Man's search for meaning.* Cutchogue, NY: Buccaneer Books.

Gramling, L., & Nugent, K. (1998). Teaching caring within the context of health. *Nurse Educator, 23*(2), 47–51. Retrieved from journals.lww.com/nurseeducatoronline/Abstract/1998/03000/Teaching _Caring_Within_the_Context_of_Health.18.aspx

Harding Clark, M. (2006). *The Lourdes hospital enquiry: An enquiry into peripartum hysterectomy at Our Lady of Lourdes Hospital, Drogheda.* Dublin, Ireland: Stationery Office.

Health Information Quality Authority. (2013). *Patient safety investigation report into services at University Hospital Galway (UHG) and as reflected in the care provided to Savita Halappanavar.* Dublin, Ireland: Author.

Health Information Quality Authority. (2015). *Report of the investigation into the safety, quality and standards of services provided by the Health Service Executive to patients in the Midland Regional Hospital, Portlaoise.* Dublin, Ireland: Author.

Health Service Executive. (2006). *Leas cross report.* Dublin, Ireland: Author.

Leininger, M. M., & Watson J. (Eds.). (1990). *The caring imperative in education.* New York, NY: National League for Nursing.

Maben, J., Latter, S., & Clark, J. M. (2007). The sustainability of ideals, values and the nursing mandate: Evidence from a longitudinal qualitative study. *Nursing Inquiry, 14*(2), 99–113. Retrieved from http://www.ncbi.nlm.nih.gov/pubmed/17518822

MacDonald-Wicks, L., & Levett-Jones T. (2012). Effective teaching of communication to health professional undergraduate and postgraduate students: A systematic review. *JBL Database of Systematic Reviews, 10*(28), 1–12. Retrieved from www.joannabriggslibrary.org/jbilibrary/index.php/jbis rir/article/view/327/532

Nursing and Midwifery Board of Ireland. (2014). *The code professional conduct and ethics for registered nurses and registered midwives.* Dublin, Ireland: Author. Retrieved from http://www.nmbi.ie/nmbi/ media/NMBI/Publications/Code-of-professional-Conduct-and-Ethics.pdf?ext=.pdf

O'Halloran, S., Wynne, M., & Cassidy, E. (2016). Position paper one: Values for nurses and midwives in Ireland, Department of Health, Dublin. Retrieved from https://www.nmbi.ie/NMBI/media/ NMBI/Position-Paper-Values-for-Nurses-and-Midwives-June-2016.pdf

Pitt, V., Powis, D., Levett-Jones, T., & Hunter, S. (2014). Nursing students' personal qualities: A descriptive study. *Nurse Education Today, 34*(9), 1196–1200. Retrieved from www.nurseeducationtoday .com/article/S0260-6917(14)00188-9/references

Roach, S. (1984). *Caring, the human mode of being: A blueprint for health professionals.* Toronto, ON, Canada: Canadian Hospital Association Press.

Royal College of Nursing. (2008). *Defending dignity: Challenges and opportunities for nursing.* London, England: Author. Retrieved from http://www.dignityincare.org.uk

Rycroft-Malone, J., Seers, K., Titchen, A., Harvey, G., Kitson, A., & McCormack, B. (2004). What counts as evidence in evidence based practice? *Journal of Advanced Nursing, 47*(1), 81–90. doi:10.1111/j.1365-2648.2004.03068.x

Tanner, C. (1990). Reflections on the curriculum revolution. *Journal of Nursing Education, 29,* 295–299. doi:10.3928/0148-4834-19900901-04

Timmins, F., Murphy, M., Caldeira, S., Ging, E., King, C., Brady, V., . . . Nolan, B. (2016). Developing agreed and accepted understandings of spirituality and spiritual care concepts among members of an innovative spirituality interest group in the Republic of Ireland. *Religions, 7*(3), 1–15. doi:10.3390/rel7030030

Timmins, F., Murphy, M., Pujol, N., Sheaf, G., Caldeira, S., Whelan, J., . . . Flanagan, B. (2016). Implementing spiritual care at the end of life in the Republic of Ireland. *European Journal of Palliative Care, 23*(1), 42–43. Retrieved from http://www.eapcnet.eu/Portals/0/Clinical/Spiritual%20care/ Publications/EJPC_23_1_Timmins.pdf

Wagner, L. A., & Seymour, M. E. (2007). A model of caring mentorship for nursing. *Journal for Nurses in Staff Development, 23,* 201–211. Retrieved from www.watsoncaringscience.org/images/features/ library/Wagner_CoachingJ_Nurs_Staff_Dev_2007.pdf

Watson, J. (1988). *Nursing: Human science and human care.* New York, NY: National League for Nursing.

Watson, J. (2005). *Caring science as sacred science.* Philadelphia, PA: F.A. Davis.

Watson, J. (2008). *Nursing: The philosophy and science of caring* (Rev. ed.). Boulder, CO: University Press of Colorado.

Watson, J. (2012). *Human caring science: A theory of nursing science and human care* (2nd ed.). Sudbury, MA: Jones & Bartlett.

Watson, J., & Smith, M. C. (2002). Caring science and the science of unitary human beings: A transtheoretical discourse for nursing knowledge development. *Journal of Advanced Nursing, 37*(5), 452–461. Retrieved from http://onlinelibrary.wiley.com/doi/10.1046/j.1365-2648.2002.02112.x/epdf

Whelan, J. (1995). *An exploratory study of the meaning and experience of caring: Staff nurses' perspectives* (Unpublished paper). University College Dublin, Ireland.

Whelan, J. (2003). *The caring dimension in nursing: A hermeneutic enquiry of students' perspectives of the meaning and experience of caring* (Unpublished master's thesis). University of Manchester, England.

# CHAPTER FIVE

# The Use of Simulation to Strengthen Humanistic Practice Among Nursing Students in the Canton of Vaud (Switzerland)

*Philippe Delmas, Otilia Froger, Muriel Harduin, Sandra Gaillard-Desmedt, and Coraline Stormacq*

## CARITAS QUOTE

*Any profession that loses its values becomes heartless; any profession that becomes heartless becomes soulless. Any profession that becomes heartless and soulless, becomes [Worthless]. (Watson, 2005, p. 44)*

*Simulation in the field of nursing education tends to focus primarily on the acquisition of clinical skills, often of a technical nature, without necessarily taking account of the uniqueness of individuals or the caring relationship. This phenomenon is all the truer in certain French-language countries where nursing is an emergent discipline. The challenge facing teaching staff remains, therefore, to construct simulation scenarios in which the* caring *relationship between the student and the standardized patient represents the focal point of the simulation session. The aim of this chapter is to share the story of a Swiss team of teachers from an institution with a long history of advocating disciplinary thought and their experience introducing a simulation activity to strengthen humanistic practice among nursing students.*

## ■ OBJECTIVES

*The objectives of this chapter are to:*

- *Describe the history and pedagogical evolution of a pioneering institution (La Source School of Nursing Science) in the development of nursing thought in Europe*

- *Identify the factors that triggered the decision by certain teachers to apply Dr. Watson's (2008, 2012) Theory of Human Caring as the foundation for developing a simulation activity*

- *Share the experience of a team of teachers in the construction and conduct of a simulation activity aimed at strengthening the caring attitudes and behaviors of nursing students*

## ■ HISTORY AND PEDAGOGICAL EVOLUTION OF NURSING SCIENCE IN EUROPE

It does not seem appropriate to expound on the integration of a nursing theory in clinical practice in French-speaking Europe without talking about the development of nursing as a discipline in Europe. In fact, the development and teaching of nursing theories often remain embryonic and depend on the particular will of institutions or groups of people. In this context, integrating Dr. Jean Watson's theoretical approach in the curriculum through practice simulation can be considered a giant step forward in undergraduate teaching methods and constitutes for our teaching staff a clear commitment to Caring Science. This progress was made possible by various factors, such as the history of the La Source School of Nursing Science and the implementation of the Bologna agreements (Council of Europe, 1999), that deserve to be highlighted for paving the way for the universitization of the nursing profession, the development of a network of French-speaking researchers interested in *caring*, and, lastly and above all, Dr. Watson's visits to La Source to conduct various colloquia. These visits, in particular, allowed members of the teaching staff to raise their own awareness of the fact that *caring* is at the core of nursing. Consequently, in order to gain a firmer grasp of the European issues related to the development of nursing science, these various factors will be covered in the following sections.

### LA SOURCE: AT THE CROSSROADS OF THE HISTORY OF NURSING THOUGHT IN THE FRENCH-SPEAKING WORLD

The history of the nursing profession and of its educational institutions has long been the preserve of the English-speaking world, which, owing to various factors such as its school system (Delmas, Sylvain, Lazure, Boudier, & Shinn, 2006), continues to be a major locus of disciplinary reflection and development. This notwithstanding, there are certain institutions in the French-speaking world, such as La Source in Lausanne, whose history and present commitment regarding the education and training of nurses have been and remain pioneers in the development of nursing thought.

Under the aegis of Valérie de Gasparin, La Source admitted its first cohort of students in 1859. It became the first international school to deliver nurse training from a purely lay perspective, 1 year before the inauguration of Florence Nightingale's school. Indeed, de Gasparin defended the idea that being a nurse was before all else a profession, just like being a teacher, and that this required a formal place where nursing could be taught outside of all religious denominations (Francillon, 2008). From its inception, the training centered on three essential points—theory, practice, and community care—and aimed to meet the needs of communities (Francillon, 2008). The community care approach remains one of the school's hallmarks, which might explain why it has been an important place of reflection on the development of nursing competencies in connection with public and community health. Despite the renewed desire by successive administrators to raise the level of nurse training, it was only with the European reform of higher education that the countries concerned committed to the Bologna Process (1999), whose mission was to harmonize the architecture of the European system of higher learning.

## THE BOLOGNA AGREEMENTS: THE LATE UNIVERSITIZATION OF THE NURSING PROFESSION IN FRENCH-SPEAKING EUROPE

The shift from vocational training to university education for nurses began in Europe around 2005 in different ways. The policy in French-speaking Switzerland was to reconsider the entire undergraduate curriculum with the emphasis placed on teaching nursing as a discipline. The first PhD holders in nursing science were recruited at the same time as the education reform was implemented, in order to raise the existing level of education through the significant contribution they would make with the knowledge they possessed of the field. It would be remiss of us if we did not talk about La Source's decades-old pedagogical culture, beginning with didactic conferences (Vienneau, 2005), before embracing socioconstructivist approaches (Vienneau, 2005); these consider learning a joint construct where individuals develop their knowledge through interactions with others. This allows for the development of narrative-based pedagogical approaches where students get the chance to reassess lived situations in a group mode and to question and share the meaning and purpose of nursing care. As pointed out by Scheckel and Ironside (2006), these approaches fostered the emergence of certain clinical concerns, which brought to light a broad array of patients' needs that would have remained unexplored under standard traditional approaches.

In recent years, expert patients living with a particular health situation have been recruited as teaching partners to help illustrate the theoretical concepts that students learn in class. These narrative activities allow them not only to develop the self-insight that enhances the capacity for knowing oneself and others but also to penetrate, with the teacher's help, someone else's world in order to gain a better understanding of what they are going through. Thus, despite its short history as a university establishment, La Source has never ceased placing the human being at the heart of its concerns, and humanist values have informed its teaching processes and content for decades. In this context, it was not surprising that Dr. Watson's (2008, 2012) Theory of Human Caring was very well received by, and even had a rallying effect on, a large portion of the teaching staff. In this connection, teaching regarding the helping relationship has been the focus of special attention on the part of the teaching staff at La Source in recent years, owing not only to changes in theoretical fundamentals flowing from exposure to continuous professional training but also to the development of international ties with the United States. The fundamentals underlying teaching of the relationship had for years remained those derived from the works of Rogers (1957). Then, contacts were established with Peplau, which led to teaching the subject based on her four phases of the interpersonal relationship: orientation, identification, exploitation, and resolution (Peplau, 1952). Continued exchanges between the teaching staff at La Source and Peplau, as well as her visit to the school, served both to enrich what and how students were taught and to stimulate teachers in their reflections, which led to the recognition that the interpersonal relationship was central to teaching and practicing nursing care.

## DR. WATSON'S VISIT TO LA SOURCE: AN EYE-OPENING AWARENESS RAISER

More recently, partnerships were created between researchers in Quebec (Drs. Cara and O'Reilly) and at La Source (Dr. Delmas) to set up a research program centered on the evaluation of an educational intervention based on the concepts of Dr. Watson's (2008, 2012) Theory of Human Caring intended for nurses working with rehabilitation and hemodialysis patients (O'Reilly, Cara, & Delmas, in press). Contacts were established between Drs. Watson, O'Reilly, and Delmas in order to organize a conference at La Source titled, *Le caring dans tous ses états: point de vue de différents acteurs* (Caring in All Its Dimensions: From the Actors' Point of View). The aim of this event was twofold: (a) confront and compare different perspectives and knowledge of the concept of *caring*, including from clinical, pedagogical, management, and philosophical angles; and (b) illustrate how the caring approach had contributed to strengthen humanist clinical practices among health professionals. Getting Dr. Watson to host the conference proved a real challenge for the staff at La Source. It was also a dream come true, as it gave them the chance to bask for a few hours in the light of an internationally renowned theorist. In her first conference at La Source, Watson placed a heavy emphasis on explaining how her theory and its concepts evolved over time and on describing the new forms of Caring Science evidence-based methods, models, and practices from the field (Watson, 2014). Certain words pronounced by Dr. Watson struck a particular chord among the teaching staff, especially the quote cited in the introduction.

These words were one of the factors that prompted us to construct a simulation activity that would put into perspective the relevance for nursing students to deploy the concepts of Dr. Watson's (2008, 2012) Theory of Human Caring in order to foster the development of a caring–healing relationship with patients. Moreover, according to Meleis (1997), the choice of a nursing theory allows strengthening the clinical practice of nurses and, a fortiori, of students by providing a structure and language that makes it possible to describe and explain clinical phenomena, to guide the action of nurses and, thus, to differentiate their practice. The various themes covered by Dr. Watson in the course of her conference at La Source bolstered the conviction among teachers that *caring* is at the core of the nursing profession and that "teaching caring becomes the moral imperative of nursing educators" (Bevis & Watson, 2000, p. 183).

## ■ APPLYING WATSON'S THEORY OF HUMAN CARING

### RELEVANCE OF THE THEORY TO THE SIMULATION ACTIVITY

The objective that the group of teachers hoped to achieve was to create an opportunity for nursing students to gain awareness, through nursing simulation, of the added benefits of developing a caring relationship with patients. The choice of Dr. Watson's (2008, 2012) Theory of Human Caring rested on various elements, including the fact that, according to Dr. Watson (2012), *caring* was at the core of nursing and nurses were vectors of caring for the patient. Under this approach, nurses and students can create a caring–healing environment through the use of intentional presence and caring connection (Herbst, 2012). According to Cara and O'Reilly (2008), the practice of *caring* seems to allow nurses to develop a value-based humanist relationship in order to alleviate human suffering and promote their dignity (Cara, 2010). To guide this practice, Dr. Watson (2008, 2012) proposed deploying 10 carative factors (CFs), whose operational application facilitates their understanding in clinical situations faced by students. Dr. Watson (1979, 1985, 1988b) has paid special attention to the development and refinement of these CFs. The factors provide a structure for studying and understanding nursing as a science of *caring*. Dr. Watson (2013) pointed out the relevance of the term *carative,* as opposed to *curative,* in order to help students mark the difference between nursing and medicine, whose primary aim is to cure the patient's disease. This element of differentiation and the CFs were, on the one hand, very useful for the development of the simulation teaching sequence and, on the other, very helpful to students, who were able to put words to their intentions, attitudes, and behaviors and, more broadly, to their vision of nursing. More specifically, there are 10 CFs in Dr. Watson's (2008, 2012) Theory of Human Caring: (a) the formation of a humanistic–altruism system of values; (b) the instillation of faith–hope; (c) the cultivation of sensitivity to one's self and to others; (d) the development of a helping–trust relationship; (e) the promotion and acceptance of the expression of positive and negative feelings; (f) the systematic use of the scientific problem-solving method for decision making; (g) the promotion of interpersonal teaching–learning; (h) the provision of a supportive, protective, and (or) corrective mental, physical, sociocultural, and spiritual environment; (i) assistance with the gratification of human needs; and (j) the allowance for existential-phenomenological forces. According to Tomey and Alligood (2002), these factors propose clear guidelines for nurse–patient interactions. As pointed out by Dr. Watson (2013), the first three factors establish the philosophical foundation for the science of *caring*. These were the factors primarily that the teaching staff took into account in constructing the simulation scenario because it appeared important to give students the opportunity, over the course of a short simulated practice activity, to shift their perspective in order to be able to grasp the human complexity of the cared-for person. Finally, certain Quebec researchers (Drs. Cara and O'Reilly) proposed a series of French documents mainly focused on the description and operationalization of the 10 CFs, which made it easier for French-speaking students to grasp the key concepts of Dr. Watson's (2008, 2012) Theory of Human Caring.

The choice of a simulation activity as a teaching sequence to permit the integration of professional *caring* in nursing was a real challenge. Indeed, Eggenberger, Keller, and Lynn (2008) pointed out that most simulation scenarios were developed in order to strengthen the students' technical skills, and thus at times reduced the quality of the nurse–patient relationship to principles of courtesy and propriety. Therefore, in the course of high-fidelity simulations, students tend to focus mostly on the acquisition of individual or group technical skills in hypertechnical care settings, thus giving a backseat to the more complex and sophisticated aspect of nursing's focus, that is, as underlined by Hills and Watson (2011): "people and inner meaning, perceptions, feelings, and the complex, relational, experiential, contextual aspect of health and healing" (p. 10). According to Eggenberger et al. (2008), students can thus become technically competent without necessarily coming into contact with patients as persons. This state of affairs can, according to Roach (2002), lead to "competence without compassion," which, in turn, can give rise to brutal and inhumane relationships between nurses and patients and culminate in a biocidic relationship between the two (Halldorsdottir, 1991). Consequently, it seemed particularly relevant to offer students a simulation activity that would allow incorporating professional *caring* in nursing simulation in order to strengthen the bioactive, if not biogenic, relationship (Halldorsdottir, 1991), or at the very least to refocus the attention of students on care centered on people rather than disease.

## Building a Simulation Scenario Incorporating the Caring Science Perspective

A simulation scenario is a clinical situation that must resemble clinical reality as much as possible. Some authors (Eggenberger et al., 2008; Webster, 2013) have proposed constructing and evaluating scenarios that place the emphasis on relational aspects of nursing care. Some scenarios have been constructed specifically on the basis of the concepts of Dr. Watson's (2008, 2012) Theory of Human Caring (Winland-Brown, Garnett, Weiss, & Newman, 2013). These authors have recommended using standardized patients because, according to Webster, Seldomridge, and Rockelli (2012), interactions between students and these patients allow the former to deploy their relational competencies in a secure environment. Thus, students invited to take part in a simulation activity can immerse themselves in a caring environment and interact with standardized patients previously trained by teachers. Within the context of this project, the situation chosen as a clinical vignette and acted out by a standardized patient involved Chantal,[1] a 33-year-old woman living with Crohn's disease who, after emergency hospitalization for an abscess, underwent surgery. Chantal was fitted with an ileostomy bag for a period of 3 months. The situation proposed to students was to meet Chantal on the third postoperative day in order to perform ostomy care. On that day, Chantal was sad. She said she was depressed and withdrawn.

The scenario was constructed on the basis of this clinical situation using a graphic algorithm that determined the attitudes and behaviors of the standardized patient according to the students' attitudes and behaviors. The teachers' intention was to give students the chance to apply caring attitudes and behaviors, such as listening, presence, respect, honesty, trust, humility, hope, and courage, in the course of their interactions with the standardized patient. Accordingly, if students in the course of the simulation centered their practice on humanist attitudes and behaviors, such as relating to Chantal as a person and not merely a patient whose bandage needed changing, paying attention to what she was living rather than to her disease, and showing respect, compassion, and listening while taking account of her needs and desires—the more the standardized patient expressed her needs, anxieties, and fears and would seek to give meaning to her experience. Conversely, in the case where students display dehumanizing attitudes and behaviors—such as focusing on her disease and technicalities (insisting on dressing the stoma as prescribed by the physician), interrupting Chantal on a regular basis, minimizing and/or generalizing her situation by treating her lived experience as normal, and giving their own advice instead of helping the person find a solution that made sense to her—the standardized patient would adopt an attitude of nonopenness, diminish if interactions with the students were not ceased, and express feelings of anger, frustration, and sadness. It is important to note that the standardized patient was expected to offer cues in the form of feelings, attitudes, and behaviors aimed at inviting students to meet her needs and relate to her on a more human

---

[1] An alias.

level when they strayed from a person-centered practice in the course of the scenario.

Once finalized, the scenario was assessed in terms of fidelity (Beydon, Dureil, & Steib, 2013), including environmental fidelity, equipment fidelity, psychological fidelity, and temporal fidelity (Jeffries, 2005, 2007, 2011). The opinions of various content and process experts were solicited. In addition, the two possible assertions of the scenario were pretested with the standardized patient and teachers. Thus, once certain aspects of fidelity had been verified, some minor adjustments were made. At this point, the scenario met the standards for simulated practice.

## ■ A SIMULATION ACTIVITY TO STRENGTHEN CARING ATTITUDES AND BEHAVIORS

### DESCRIPTION OF THE DIFFERENT STAGES OF THE SIMULATION ACTIVITY

Jeffries (2005, 2007) and Demaurex and Vu (2013) have proposed that simulation sessions should be conducted according to four stages: briefing, implementation, debriefing, and conclusion. At each stage, different aspects must be taken into account, including objectives and planning, fidelity/realism, level of complexity, participant support, and debriefing structure. In addition, the teachers at La Source demonstrated creativity by initiating complementary periods of prepreparation, which included reflective practice exercises for students prior to the simulation session.

### PREPARING STUDENTS TO EXPERIENCE A CARING RELATIONSHIP

In order to facilitate the sharing of experiences during the simulation session, 1 week prior to the activity, second-year undergraduate students were invited to complete reflective practice exercises in which they had to write down a significant care or personal situation that they had experienced and reassess it from the perspective of Watson's (2008, 2012) Theory of Human Caring. To guide them in this analysis, the teachers proposed that they relate the highlights of their professional or personal experience to the 10 CFs. To facilitate this exercise, the teachers provided them with the French-language version (EIIP-70; Cossette, Cara, Ricard, & Pepin, 2005) of the Caring Nurse–Patient Interaction Scale (CNPI-70), which describes caring attitudes and behaviors in relation to the 10 CFs proposed by Dr. Watson (1979, 1988a). This instrument was meant to help students self-assess how often they expressed caring attitudes/behaviors in the course of their professional or personal experience. Furthermore, the students were encouraged to develop their self-insight by completing mindfulness exercises that were accessible online. As a result, during the briefing period with the students, which is described in the following text, a discussion could be had between them and the teachers regarding their understanding of the 10 CFs in relation to their experiences. Though such a reflective stage prior to scenario implementation has not been developed much within the context of traditional simulation-based learning, it appeared indispensable to the teaching staff for creating a caring environment and contributing to the development of a caring practice, which was one of the objectives of the simulation activity.

## Briefing

This is a key moment prior to the implementation stage where teachers and students meet in the simulation environment. The teachers' ultimate objective here is to create a climate of trust, security, and sharing, which are essential elements of an environment conducive to the development of transpersonal relationships. In order to foster this caring environment, students were invited to complete mindfulness exercises. These lasted 5 minutes and were intended to help students sharpen their self-insight and, therefore, to be better prepared to meet a person in a human-to-human relationship. Self-centeredness is a key element for students to be able to identify their own thoughts and emotions and to adopt the right disposition for observing them without being tempted to downplay them or to brush them away. In short, the students were prepared for the purpose of scrutinizing their own thoughts, feelings, and sensations. Then, the teachers revisited the significant situations encountered by the students in the course of clinical practicums and facilitated the process of tying the experiences described and lived by the students in practice settings together with the CFs deployed. This moment of sharing allowed the students to gain a better grasp of the importance of caring attitudes and behaviors in daily practice as the foundation of the sort of humanistic care that each and every member of humanity should be entitled to. At the end of this period of exchange came the moment of briefing immediately before the simulated practice. This stage served to contextualize the meeting for the participants. It consisted primarily of reading out the clinical vignette to introduce the simulation scenario (Demaurex & Vu, 2013), which, in our case, was Chantal's situation. Other elements were added by the teachers, such as an analysis of Chantal's situation in the light of how she might experience it and how the students might develop their listening, presence, and respect in her regard, as well as instill hope. This preparation before the meeting served to awaken in the students a knowledge of self and others as *caring*. Then, each teacher accompanying a group of 10 students solicited one student to play the role of the nurse who is to meet Chantal to deliver postoperative care.

## Implementation: Encountering Chantal

The encounter between the student and Chantal constituted the core of this simulated practice. During the analysis of the different simulated practice sequences by the teachers, a certain degree of homogeneousness in how the interactions between the students and Chantal unfolded over time appears. Indeed, in the early moments of the encounter, most of the students called upon the scientific and theoretical knowledge required for Chantal's postoperative clinical management in order to address her pharmacological and physiological needs (vital signs measurement, pain assessment, information). From the point of view of the fundamental patterns of knowing described by Carper (1978), it can be hypothesized that the students deployed knowledge derived primarily from empirical patterns of knowing. Then, the students developed a more subjective analysis of the situation and swung back and forth between a narrower and a wider viewpoint. This was akin to the *alternating rhythms* described by Mayeroff (1971), which, according to Boykin and Schoenhofer (2013), provide an approach to applying caring empirical knowledge. Simultaneously, the students focused on the inherent meaning of the situation experienced by Chantal through an authentic presence and acceptance of the other person as a human being living a particular health situation. They established a relationship of trust with Chantal, in which it was possible for both persons to voice feelings, lived experiences, and doubts without being judged by the other. In other words, the students very quickly applied caring personal knowledge (Boykin & Schoenhofer, 2013) in order to establish a therapeutic relationship that allowed Chantal to find meaning in the experience she was living. Finally, throughout the encounter with Chantal, the teachers underscored that, in the course of these interactions, the students reinforced their engagement to care for Chantal and their respect for her right to self-determination, which bears witness to a certain ethical stance on the part of the students and, by the same token, to the deployment of ethical knowledge (Carper, 1978).

## Debriefing

Debriefing took place right after the simulated practice. It is seen as a reflective thought session that allows the students to evaluate their actions, decisions, mode of communication, and capacity to deal with the unexpected in a secure universe where mistakes are permitted (Dieckmann, Reddersen, Zieger, & Rall, 2008; Haskvitz & Koop, 2004; Jeffries, 2005; Mort & Donahue, 2004). In our case, the teacher, the students who observed the simulated practice, the student who took part in the simulated practice, and the standardized patient came together to share their experience and understanding of the situation. In order to facilitate dialogue and evaluation among the different parties, the teacher organized the debriefing session into the following three phases as recommended by Savoldelli and Boet (2013): reaction (expressing of emotions), analysis (setting in motion the reflective process), and summary (brief recap to close the session). During the reaction phase, the teacher again used the mindfulness exercises to help participants focus on the present and examine their thoughts and feelings without judging. The aim here was to help participants awaken to experience and gain a higher degree of mindfulness. During the analysis phase, the teacher asked the participants to identify, using the French-language version (EIIP-70; Cossette et al., 2005) of the CNPI-70, the caring attitudes and behaviors deployed by the student in the course of the simulated practice and those that they would recommend adopting were they to care for Chantal. Based on the results obtained by the participants, the teacher next asked them to compare and share their points of view beginning with the self-evaluation of the student who played the role of the nurse. The precise descriptors provided by the EIIP-70/CNPI-70 facilitated the reflective process and the organization of one's thoughts at the time of sharing. Thus, confronting and comparing points of view allowed gaining a better grasp of the nature of the interactions that the student implemented in the course of the simulated practice from the perspective of the 10 CFs. The capacity to put words to and make connections between theory and practice allowed the students to acquire a deeper appreciation for the uniqueness of nursing care. Moreover, the standardized patient added considerably to the quality of the debriefing by sharing her feelings and her own perception of the quality of the relationship with the student. This open dialogue allowed all the participants to better understand the impact that the caring attitudes and behaviors, deployed by a nurse, can have on the quality of life of a vulnerable person. The teacher closed this debriefing phase with a series of questions concerning how the simulation session might be improved.

## ■ CONCLUSION

Though often employed to learn clinical skills of a technical nature, simulation appears relevant to facilitate the integration of concepts derived from a nursing theory such as Watson's (2008, 2012) Theory of Human Caring. As discussed by Eggenberger et al. (2008), simulation activities are rarely reported in the field of Caring Science, but these need to be developed. Indeed, practical experimentation in a secure setting allows students to make the connection between theory and practice. This is a key method to help nursing students integrate complex phenomena into clinical practice. In this context, simulation plays a major role. Finally, the acquisition of a distinct vocabulary by nursing students through simulation activities is another important outcome worth highlighting. This allows naming elements of analysis and intervention in a distinct manner, thus differentiating the specific contribution of nursing care to the health of patients and, more broadly, to that of the population. Finally, facilitating the integration of Dr. Watson's (2008, 2012) Theory of Human Caring in the students' curriculum also constitutes a political act, equipping nursing students with a body of knowledge, know-how, and interpersonal skills that is specific to them, thereby giving visibility to their care acts and, by extension, to their profession. It has never been more urgent for each profession to identify the value proposition for the health of populations than in today's global economy where the dominant discourse is centered on rationality and profit. This is why it is an ethical and philosophical imperative that *caring* be recognized as the nursing profession that has the most to offer in the way of added value.

## ■ REFERENCES

Bevis, E. O., & Watson, J. (2000). *Toward a caring curriculum: A new pedagogy for nursing*. Boston, MA: Jones & Bartlett.

Beydon, L., Dureil, B., & Steib, A. (2013). Place de la simulation dans la rectification des professionnels de la santé [Using simulation to rectify the practice of health professionals]. In S. Boet, J. C. Grangy, & G. Savoldelli (Eds.), *La simulation en santé: de la théorie à la pratique* (pp. 267–276). Paris, France: Springer.

Boykin, A., & Schoenhofer, S. (2013). Caring in nursing: Analysis of extant theory. In M. C. Smith, M. C. Turkel, & Z. Robinson Wolf (Eds.), *Caring in nursing classics: An essential resource* (pp. 33–42). New York, NY: Springer Publishing.

Cara, C. (2010). Les fondements théoriques du Caring dans la pratique infirmière [The theoretical fundamentals of caring in nursing practice]. In P. Potter & A. Perry (Eds.), *Soins infirmiers: Théorie et pratique* (pp. 84–99). Montréal, QC, Canada: Chenelière Éducation.

Cara, C., & O'Reilly, L. (2008). S'approprier la théorie du Human Caring de Jean Watson par la pratique réflexive lors d'une situation clinique [Grasping Jean Watson's Theory of Human Caring through reflective practice in a clinical situation]. *Recherche en soins infirmiers, 95*, 37–45.

Carper, B. (1978). Fundamental patterns of knowing in nursing. *Advanced Nursing Science, 1*(1), 13–24.

Cossette, S., Cara, C., Ricard, N., & Pepin, J. (2005). Assessing nurse-patient interactions from a caring perspective: Report of the development and preliminary psychometric testing of the caring nurse-patient interactions scale. *International Journal of Nursing Studies, 42*(6), 673–686. doi:10.1016/j.ijnurstu.2004.10.004

Council of Europe. (1999). The European higher education area: The Bologna Declaration of 19 June 1999—Joint declaration of the European Ministers of Education. Bologna, Italy: Author.

Delmas, P., Sylvain, H., Lazure, G., Boudier, C., & Shinn, T. (2006). Le développement des savoirs disciplinaires: une histoire d'institution: approche de Joseph Ben David [Developing disciplinary knowledge: Joseph Ben David's approach]. *Perspective soignante, 26*, 103–120.

Demaurex, F., & Vu, N. V. (2013). Séance de simulation avec patient standardisé [Standardized patient simulation sessions]. In S. Boet, J. C. Grangy, & G. Savoldelli (Eds.), *La simulation en santé: de la théorie à la pratique* (pp. 303–312). Paris, France: Springer.

Dieckmann, P., Reddersen, S., Zieger, J., & Rall, M. (2008). Video-assisted debriefing in simulation-based training of crisis resource management. In R. Kyle & B. Murray (Eds.), *Clinical simulation* (pp. 667–676). Amsterdam, The Netherlands: Elsevier.

Eggenberger, T. R., Keller, K. B., & Lynn, C. E. (2008). Grounding nursing simulations in caring: An innovative approach. *International Journal of Human Caring, 12*(2), 42–46.

Francillon, D. (2008). *Enjeux et dynamique de la formation des gardes-malades à celle de soins infirmiers. Une école-hôpital: la Source 1859–1977. Rapport de recherche* [Issues and dynamics: From home nurse training to nursing care training. La Source teaching hospital from 1859 to 1977. Research report]. Lausanne, Switzerland: Institut et Haute Ecole de la Santé La Source.

Halldorsdottir, S. (1991). Five basic modes of being with another. In D. A. Gaut & M. Leininger (Eds.), *Caring: The compassionate healer* (pp. 37–49). New York, NY: National League for Nursing.

Haskvitz, L. M., & Koop, E. C. (2004). Students struggling in clinical? A new role for the patient simulator. *Journal of Nursing Education, 43*(4), 181–184. doi:10.3928/01484834-20040401-06

Herbst, A. (2012). Impact of intentional caring behaviors on nurse's perceptions of caring in the workplace, nurses' intent to stay, and patients' perceptions of being cared for. In J. Nelson & J. Watson (Eds.), *Measuring caring: International research on Caritas as healing* (pp. 173–194). New York, NY: Springer Publishing.

Hills, M., & Watson, J. (2011). *Creating a caring science curriculum: An emancipatory pedagogy for nursing*. New York, NY: Springer Publishing.

Jeffries, P. R. (2005). A framework for designing, implementing, and evaluating simulations used as teaching strategies in nursing. *Nursing Education Perspectives, 26*(2), 96–103.

Jeffries, P. R. (2007). *Simulation in nursing education: From conceptualization to evaluation.* New York, NY: National League for Nursing.

Jeffries, P. R. (2011, June). *State of the science in simulation: The simulation framework.* Communication presented at the 10th Annual International Nursing Simulation/Learning Resource Center Conference, Orlando, FL.

Mayeroff, M. (1971). *On caring.* New York, NY: HarperCollins.

Meleis, A. I. (1997). *Theorical nursing: Development & progress* (3rd ed.). Philadelphia, PA: Lippincott Williams & Wilkins.

Mort, T. C., & Donahue, S. P. (2004). Debriefing: The basics. In W. F. Dunn (Ed.), *Simulation in critical care and beyond* (pp. 76–83). Des Plaines, IL: Society of Critical Care Medicine.

O'Reilly, L., Cara, C., & Delmas, P. (2016). Developing an educational intervention to strengthen the humanistic practices of hemodialysis nurses in Switzerland. *International Journal of Human Caring, 20*(1), 25–30.

Peplau, H. E. (1952). *Interpersonal relations in nursing, a conceptual frame of reference for psychodynamic nursing.* New York, NY: Putnam.

Roach, S. (2002). *Caring, the human mode of being* (2nd ed.). Ottawa, ON, Canada: CHA Press.

Rogers, C. R. (1957). The necessary and sufficient conditions for therapeutic personality change. *Journal of Consulting Psychology, 21*(2), 95–103. doi:10.1037/h0045357

Savoldelli, G., & Boet, S. (2013). Séance de simulation: du briefing au débriefing [Simulation sessions: From briefing to debriefing]. In S. Boet, J. C. Grangy, & G. Savoldelli (Eds.), *La simulation en santé: de la théorie à la pratique* (pp. 313–328). Paris, France: Springer.

Scheckel, M. M., & Ironside, P. M. (2006). Cultivating interpretive thinking through enacting narrative pedagogy. *Nursing Outlook, 54*(3), 159–165. doi:10.1016/j.outlook.2006.02.002

Tomey, A. M., & Alligood, M. R. (2002). *Nursing theorists and their work* (5th ed.). Philadelphia, PA: Mosby/Elsevier Health Science.

Vienneau, R. (2005). *Apprentissage et enseignement: Théories et pratiques* [Learning and teaching: Theories and practices]. Montréal, QC, Canada: Gaëtan Morin.

Watson, J. (1979). *Nursing: The philosophy and science of caring.* Boston, MA: Little Brown.

Watson, J. (1985). *Nursing: Human science and human care.* Norwalk, CT: Appleton-Century-Crofts.

Watson, J. (1988a). New dimensions of human caring theory. *Nursing Science Quarterly, 1*(4), 175–181.

Watson, J. (1988b). *Nursing: Human science and human care. A theory of nursing* (2nd printing). New York, NY: National League for Nursing.

Watson, J. (2005). *Caring Science as sacred science.* Philadelphia, PA: F.A. Davis.

Watson, J. (2008). *Nursing: The philosophy and science of caring* (Rev. ed.). Boulder, CO: University Press of Colorado.

Watson, J. (2012). *Human caring science: A theory of nursing* (2nd ed.). Sudbury, MA: Jones & Bartlett.

Watson, J. (2013). Nursing: The philosophy and science of caring. In M. C. Smith, M. C. Turkel, & Z. Robinson Wolf (Eds.), *Caring in nursing classics. An essential resource* (pp. 143–153). New York, NY: Springer Publishing.

Watson, J. (2014). *Caring science as disciplinary foundation of nursing and health care: Returning to heart.* Communication presented at the first "Colloque multidisciplinaire francophone: La pratique humaniste dans tous ses états: Point de vue de différents acteurs du soin," Lausanne, Switzerland.

Webster, D. (2013). Promoting therapeutic communication and patient-centered care using standardized patients. *Journal of Nursing Education, 52*(11), 645–648. doi:10.3928/01484834-2013 1014-06

Webster, D., Seldomridge, L., & Rockelli, L. (2012). Making it real: Using standardized patients to bring case studies to life. *Journal of Psychosocial Nursing and Mental Health Services, 50*(5), 36–41. doi:10.3928/02793695-20120410-06

Winland-Brown, J. E., Garnett, S., Weiss, J., & Newman, D. (2013). Using the six Cs as a caring tool to evaluate the simulation experience. *International Journal of Human Caring, 17*(2), 9–15.

# PART THREE

# Caritas Enlightened Leadership

Caritas enlightened leadership is an emerging style of leadership that is informed by the Theory of Human Caring and the 10 Caritas Processes. It is a values-based leadership that rests on the philosophical–moral–ethical stance of caring that goes beyond ego-self by inspiring a collective Caritas consciousness in a higher vibrational frequency field. Caritas enlightened leadership rests on a relational ontology that can influence persons, systems, and the world. Dr. Patrick Palmieri, a Peruvian American Caring Scholar living in Peru, leverages his background in health care leadership and nursing to develop nursing leadership and advance the discipline in Peru. This pioneer–innovator, who was instrumental in starting a professional nursing organization in Peru, is evolving the Caritas consciousness through collaboration with Dr. Watson. Dr. Sara Horton-Deutsch, the Watson Caring Science Endowed Chair at the College of Nursing, University of Colorado Denver, reveals how she has evolved caring leadership tenets through conceptual scholarship and research. Dr. Jacqueline Somerville, chief nursing officer at Brigham and Women's Hospital in Boston, Massachusetts, chronicles her hospital's journey to becoming a Watson Caring Science Affiliate, specifically relating to creating intentionality and heart-centered leaders.

# CHAPTER SIX

# Thinking, Acting, and Leading Through Caring Science Literacy

Sara Horton-Deutsch

## CARITAS QUOTE

*When nursing individually and collectively engages in caring healing practices at this higher-deeper, subtle but powerful vibratory level, we will turn to words and actions that vibrate at a higher level—words and actions that nurture Spirit and the human soul of our work. (Watson, 2008, p. 199)*

*This chapter shares my journey from a scholar of mindful-awareness and reflective practice to an expanded leadership role through the integration of Caring Science. I begin by sharing the tenets of my work that align with Caring Science and then explore how this connects with my leadership journey. Next, I explore some of the latest research on leadership and how these bodies of work align with Caring Science and Caritas Literacy. This section aims to demonstrate how Caring Science Theory guides my thinking while the language of Caring Science provides a way to demonstrate congruency between thinking and actions through the use of high-energy words demonstrating literacy. Finally, I share tenets of caring leadership and encourage others to reflect on their own vision of caring leadership as well as the words, actions, and practices that embody it.*

## ■ OBJECTIVES

*The objectives of this chapter are to:*
- *Chronicle the personal/professional journey to Caritas leadership*
- *Synthesize current findings in caring leadership*
- *Introduce tenets of Caritas leadership*

## ■ JOURNEY TO CARING SCIENCE AND CARITAS

My first recollection of Caring Science was through a lecture and readings from my undergraduate nursing theory course. We were asked to write a paper about a theory that resonated with us. Of course, I chose Jean Watson's philosophy and science of care. I suspect this was more a case of the theory finding me than of me finding it.

I was raised in the midwestern United States in a family of professional caregivers who treated the whole person in a relational way. For instance, as a child during my summer vacation, I recall going on home visits with my grandfather who was a small town physician. He would sit down beside the bed with the patient and take as much time as was needed. Afterward, we would often sit on the porch and drink iced tea with the family caregiver before leaving. Sometimes we would come home with pecans or vegetables fresh from the garden as a means of payment for his services. Although a student in a U.S. nursing school, I completed my community health nursing in Grantham, England. My preceptor, a health visitor, and I would call on patients in their homes for the entire day. We often carried in firewood and then prepared and drank hot tea with the patient as a way to set the stage for a meaningful visit. This approach to caring and health demonstrated presence, honored the whole person, and set the stage for opening up to and responding to the unique needs of the person. I did not realize it at the time, but these experiences were the embodiment of Caring Science.

## ■ KEY ELEMENTS OF CARING SCIENCE, CARITAS, AND CARITAS LITERACY

Over the past decade, most of my scholarship has been in mindful-awareness and reflective practice. This work closely aligns with the tenets of Caring Science and caring literacy including vulnerability, self-care, and authentic presence.

### MINDFUL-AWARENESS AND REFLECTIVE PRACTICE

Creating space to nurture our inner selves and thoughtfully consider our responses to others is supported through the condition of stillness and an opening to the practice of mindfulness. Mindfulness is paying attention, in the moment, on purpose, and without judgment (Kabat-Zinn, 1990). It allows for an expanded awareness and the courage to observe oneself with an open mind and heart. Mindful-awareness interweaves intentionality, attention, and attitude (Shapiro, Carlson, Astin, & Freedman, 2006). These are all qualities of caring consciousness that allow us to see not only what a person is now but also what he or she may become or is becoming (Watson, 2008). These qualities are all part of a personal and professional journey of the nurse (Watson, 2005) and are nurtured by mindful-awareness and through reflective practices.

Reflective practices include any type of attentive consideration, including thinking, contemplation, or meditation, which helps us to make sense of our actions and leads to meaning, understanding, growth, and transformation (Horton-Deutsch, 2012). Reflection helps us to develop a capacity for openness, whole-heartedness, and responsibility (Dewey, 1933). It supports deep learning where our understandings come to the surface and foster growth. It involves learning from everyday experiences with an aim to realize a desirable practice (Johns, 2004, 2006). These practices are both deliberate and intuitive and can take place before, during, and/or after encounters with others. They encourage person-centered care, support collaboration and open communication, and foster a culture of safety. They also promote the development of self-awareness, interpersonal relationships, and emotionally competent leaders (Horton-Deutsch, 2012; Horton-Deutsch & Sherwood, 2008).

## VULNERABILITY

From 2008 through 2011, I had the privilege of working with doctoral student Kristen Lombard at Indiana University. Kristen was interested in nurses' experiences of PeerSpirit Circle—a nonhierarchical, intentional, and relationship-centered practice of collaboration—and its potential impact on nursing practice, education, and research, as well as the evolution of the profession and health care (Lombard, 2011). From this phenomenological research, Kristen unearthed the value of intentional preparation of interpersonal space for safe human interaction, creating a sacred space where members are free to be vulnerable and engage in genuine dialogue, and through this experience reconnect with deeper humanity.

In Lombard's (2011) study, nurses shared their fear of being vulnerable as an obstacle to creating and allowing space. Nurses explained the need to fill, measure, and conquer space, allowing them to avoid feeling uncomfortable and vulnerable. Lombard suggested that a model of practice that creates safe spaces allows for the expression of vulnerabilities, creating stronger collaboration. Similarly, Wiklund Gustin and Wagner (2012) explored nursing teachers' understanding of self-compassion as a source to compassionate care. They found that respect for human vulnerability preserved dignity and that respect was an important part for helping–trusting relationships and for creating a healing environment. The challenge for health care professionals is that our culture has little tolerance for vulnerability

(Brown, 2010). For example, we have been conditioned to avoid and eliminate suffering. At the same time, it is part of the human experience and is inescapable. However, according to research, vulnerability is a strong ally for survival and is a strength that leads to new awareness, inviting a new level of sureness and courage to manifest (Brown, 2012; Lombard & Horton-Deutsch, 2012). According to Brown (2012), vulnerability is the core of all emotions and feelings; it is the birthplace of love, belonging, joy, courage, empathy, and creativity. It is the source of hope, empathy, accountability, and authenticity. Allowing vulnerability can call us to a willingness to be in a space of not knowing and authenticity. "It allows a human-to-human connection that expands our compassion and caring and keeps alive our common humanity" (Watson, 2008, p. 5). Allowing vulnerability has the potential to bring us to a higher level of consciousness where suffering is less, and allows us to make use and meaning of the suffering in our and others lives.

## SELF-CARE

When we have a perception of no space, time, or energy for openness and vulnerability, we risk losing our capacity to nurture relationships with ourselves and others. As nurses, we frequently talk about the importance of self-care and nurturing relationships but have little idea of how to do it. It is not uncommon for nurses to report the experience of nurturing self or being nurtured by others as feeling uncomfortable, because we find ourselves in a position of feeling vulnerable. Yet, how can we teach others how to nurture and care for self, if we do not know how to do it? Importantly, how do we learn to receive nurturing and care from others? Through mindful and reflective practices, we become aware of uncomfortable thoughts and feelings. This awareness is the first step in reflection. Being open and curious to our emotions can encourage more exploration and discovery, leading to more self-awareness (Horton-Deutsch, Drew, & Beck-Coon, 2012). Moment-to-moment awareness and presence are about paying attention to self and others. This form of mindfulness allows us to bear witness to our own suffering and respond with kindness and understanding. This then allows us to enhance our own self-care and caring for others. Mindfulness is a form of self-care that uses systematic and routine approaches to promote one's physical, spiritual, and emotional well-being.

## AUTHENTIC PRESENCE

Authentic presence has been defined as the practice of genuineness, the ability to self-reflect, being in the moment, offering caring communication, and being honest with oneself and others (Lombard & Horton-Deutsch, 2012). Presence is a skill that is essential to caring in a way that connects with and embraces the spirit of the other. It requires full attention to the here and now, and conveys a concern for the inner life and personal meaning of another (Sitzman & Watson, 2014). This form of caring—transpersonal caring—is a deeper form that appreciates we are all connected and what affects one of us, in some way, affects the other. It is as much about our way of being with another person as what we are doing for him or her.

The German philosopher Hans-Georg Gadamer (1996) describes authentic presence as an embodied manifestation of mindfulness. When nurses bring their full selves into the moment, they bring this full wakefulness into the space that can then be shared. Space, the birthplace of mindfulness, is a place to practice authentic presence to self and others (Lombard & Horton-Deutsch, 2012). Providing space and being authentically present is an act of caring. It is the birthplace of faith, hope, healing, and wholeness. It allows us to enter the inner life-world of self/other (Watson, 2008).

## ■ KEY ELEMENTS OF MY LEADERSHIP JOURNEY

My first formal study of leadership began in 2007 when I was asked to teach a graduate-level course on the subject. I was introduced to Tim Porter-O'Grady and Kathy Malloch's text *Quantum Leadership* (2007). While reading their book, I began to appreciate the complexity of leadership and the inner work that is required to be an effective leader. It was the first time I considered the value of concepts like vulnerability, risk taking, and authenticity as key ingredients to be successful as a leader.

Knowing I wanted to be a leader with courage, compassion, and consciousness, I decided to engage in the inner work of leadership during my sabbatical in 2012. I found the Leadership Circle Profile 360° Feedback Assessment and Coaching Certification to be the most comprehensive work on leadership development. Ten colleagues provided feedback and then I completed a self-assessment to determine my creative competencies and reactive tendencies. This assessment provided me with a deeper understanding of myself, the world, and my relationship to others. This deeper awareness aided in understanding the interaction between inner assumptions and outer behaviors. To this day, I pull out my profile (graphically displayed in a circle) to gain insights and to see the whole picture. This work has recently been published in a first textbook and is a fully integrated model of leadership (Anderson & Adams, 2016). The creative competencies in this profile that are consistent with Caring Science and literacy include self-awareness, relating, authenticity, and systems awareness.

## ■ HOW I HAVE IMPLEMENTED THE THEORY IN MY WORK

While I always knew the principles of mindful-awareness and reflective practices were an important component of Caring Science, it was not until I entered the Caritas Coach Education Program (CCEP) in the fall of 2013 that I realized that while I was not always using the language of Caring Science, my body–mind–spirit was that of a Caritas nurse. Looking back, it was an important revelation; the thought of fully embodying Caring Science through Caritas Literacy was a way to deepen my existing scholarship and practices as a caring leader. "The opportunity to study, research, explore, identify, describe, express and question the relation and intersection between and among the ethical, ontological, epistemological, method-ological, pedagogical, and praxis aspects of nursing, including health policies and administrative practices . . . provides the opportunity to seek congruence between and among nursing, humanities, the arts, and human subject matter and phenom-ena of caring knowledge and practices" (Watson, 2008, p. 22).

The discovery of Caring Science and its language has been a profound awakening—speaking to who I am, what I am to be. Martin Luther King expressed the importance of the use of language (words) when he asked us to consider whether our words are used to inspire or to shame, or whether we use our words to wel-come and invite or to intimidate. The theory of Caring Science guides my think-ing while the language of Caring Science provides a way to demonstrate congru-ency between thinking and actions through the use of high-energy words. Clarity comes from taking action by mindfully using words that positively energize myself and others.

Since becoming the Watson Caring Science Endowed Chair at the College of Nursing, University of Colorado Denver in December of 2013, I have sought to clarify my role and discover the best way to lead the Watson Caring Science Center as I work in partnership with Dr. Watson and her Watson Caring Sci-ence Institute. I readily discovered that the theory, practices, and language of Caring Science are very different from, and often in conflict with, the practices and languages of a system of higher education that is becoming more and more corpo-rate/bureaucratic; the former emphasizing transformation, whereas the latter trans-action. I often struggle with what is being asked of me at this time. What steps do I need to take to get to the other side of these challenges? How can I bridge these seemingly competing perspectives to positively influence health care, healing, and humanity?

Reflecting on these questions, I revisited my qualitative research with col-leagues on becoming a nurse faculty leader (Horton-Deutsch et al., 2014; Horton-Deutsch, Young, & Nelson, 2010; Pardue, Young, Horton-Deutsch, Pearsall, & Halstead, n. d.; Young, Pardue, & Horton-Deutsch, 2015; Young, Pearsall, Stiles, Nelson, & Horton-Deutsch, 2011); reviewed some of the latest global research and scholarship on leadership (Kouzes & Posner, 2012); examined more closely the disciplines perspective on mindful leadership (Johns, 2016); and further reflected on how these bodies of work come together with Caring Science to fur-ther my practice as a leader. Finally, I identified a series of practices that allow me to work through the challenges of competing paradigms (caring/holistic vs. bureaucratic/corporate). They are inclusive of the Caritas Processes and Caritas Literacy and are applied to the thoughts and actions of caring leaders.

## BECOMING A NURSE FACULTY LEADER

Over the past 9 years, a number of nursing faculty from colleges/universities across the United States and I have engaged in a series of interpretative qualitative studies of the lived experience of becoming nurse faculty leaders. The initial study findings were published in 2011, explicating the major themes of advancing reform, being thrust into leadership, taking risks, and facing challenges (Young et al., 2011), while subgroups of the team published individual themes that were interpreted in greater depth (Horton-Deutsch et al., 2010, 2014; Pardue et al., manuscript in preparation; Pearsall et al., 2014; Stiles, Pardue, Young, & Morales, 2011). Underpinning the collective work was the practice of reflecting on one's experience; the cumulative findings from the series of studies on the practices of becoming a nurse faculty leader illuminated the importance of reflective skills (Young et al., 2015).

What I learned from this series of studies was the value of reflection as an intentional strategy for leadership development. Stories from nurse faculty leaders illuminated how advancing reform, being thrust into leadership, and taking risks and facing challenges are familiar leadership experiences that require thorough and thoughtful examination. Reflection serves to enhance understanding, refine personal skill, and facilitate the complex landscape of leadership.

In alignment with the principles of Caring Science, these leadership practices facilitate self-exploration; thoughtful interactions with self and others, that is, caring literacy; and values clarification. More specifically, self- and other-awareness, active listening, and relating to others in new ways aligns with the Caritas Processes and caring literacy practices of presence and equanimity with self and others, allowing for expression of positive and negative feelings, and learning within the context of a caring relationship by staying within the other's frame of reference.

## GLOBAL RESEARCH AND SCHOLARSHIP ON LEADERSHIP

Through our work on leadership, my colleagues and I have frequently turned to the evidence-based work of Kouzes and Posner (2003, 2007, 2012) to validate our findings. With each new edition of their book, they update their research and integrate it with findings from other scholars. What remains consistent is that when leaders do their best, they engage in five practices: model the way, inspire a shared vision, challenge the process, enable others to act, and encourage the heart.

Simply stated, leadership is not about who you are but rather about what you do (Kouzes & Posner, 2012). Language matters, given that much of what we do is expressed through language. Their work further suggests that our behavior is what earns us respect as leaders. "Exemplary leaders know that if they want to gain commitment and achieve the highest standards, they must be models of the behavior they expect of others" (Kouzes & Posner, 2012, p. 16). In other words, they must model the way, be clear about their principles, and clarify these values through their voice. They emphasize that words and deeds must be consistent and the way to make them explicit is by aligning actions with shared values. This approach emphasizes leading by example over command.

Next, leaders inspire a shared vision by imagining and enabling possibilities, as well as creating something new. Equally important, leaders must be able to connect to the past, to the history of the organization. What I found most important was that commitment must be inspired; it cannot be commanded. There must be a unity of purpose that comes from demonstrating an understanding of followers' needs and having their interests at heart. When this unity of purpose or shared vision is expressed from the heart, with enthusiasm and passion, it is simultaneously ignited in others.

I have often found myself struggling with how to transform the way things are done in the "academy," where the system is frequently fraught with policies, procedures, rituals, and traditions. Kouzes and Posner (2012) remind me that the best leaders employ the third practice of leadership through challenging the status quo. No one becomes his or her personal best by keeping things the same. Becoming our personal best often requires overcoming uncertainty and fear. As leaders, we must venture out and make something happen. Similar to what my colleagues and I found in our research on becoming a nurse faculty leader (Horton-Deutsch et al., 2014; Pearsall et al., 2014), innovation comes from experimenting and taking risks. And when we take risks, failures will occur. However, by working together, taking small steps, and learning along the way, we can also increase our likelihood of generating small wins. Simply stated, Kouzes and Posner (2012) emphasize that the best leaders are also the best learners. Caring Science encompasses these principles through the emphasis on creative problem solving and solution seeking, staying with others' frame of reference while simultaneously shifting toward an expanded view.

Next, Kouzes and Posner's (2012) fourth practice of exemplary leaders is enabling others to act. No dream becomes reality and transforms the way we do things through the actions of one person. Exemplary leaders build trust and value strong relationships with others. They take the time to build personal relationships, treat everyone with respect, and openly communicate. They simultaneously give others a voice, building team collaboration and individual accountability. By trusting others . . . others begin to trust us. Our colleagues work at their best when they feel empowered, independent, and connected. By engaging in this way, leaders build new leaders. Similarly, Caring Science is rooted in trusting–caring relationships that encourage the expression of feelings and thoughtful actions.

Finally, exemplary leaders encourage the heart through genuine acts of caring. Recognizing others and showing appreciation helps to move individuals and teams forward. Done genuinely, it creates a spirit of community. It is a place to demonstrate how behaviors are aligned with our values. When it comes from the heart, these caring acts build a sense of collective identity and community that can carry a group through extraordinary tough times (Kouzes & Posner, 2012). Interestingly, this fifth practice of leadership is where Caring Science begins with an emphasis on loving-kindness, compassion, and equanimity with self and others.

For over a decade, Kouzes and Posner (2003, 2007, 2012) have demonstrated how these five practices make a difference in commitment and performance. One of the things I find most profound from their research is that workplace engagement and commitment are significantly explained by how the leader behaves and not by any particular characteristic of the constituents. So how we behave as leaders is the most important aspect of our work. If we want to have a significant impact on others, on organizations, and on communities, we must engage in caring acts, demonstrated through caring literacy and caring practices.

Kouzes and Posner's (2003, 2007, 2012) work aligns beautifully with Caring Science and my understanding of caring leadership. It involves lifelong learning through experience, whereas I aim for more desirable, effective, and satisfying experiences, whether in personal or professional endeavors. It focuses on caring acts and taking responsibility, and as a leader modeling the way for others. It includes using authentic dialogue, inspiring others to be adventurous and take risks, remaining open to feedback, building and sustaining a compassionate community, and leading from the heart. Their work validates my own values about leadership and is in alignment with the Caritas Processes.

## A DISCIPLINARY PERSPECTIVE ON LEADERSHIP

The most recent work that has influenced my thinking on how to think, act, and become a caring leader comes from Christopher Johns' book *Mindful Leadership* (2016). Having just been published, it was like coming full circle in my own journey. I have studied and built on Johns' work on reflective practice for over a decade. He is once again guiding me toward the type of leader I want to become. Johns (2016, p. 29) offers the following definition of leadership: "Leadership is mindful, insightful and caring, ever vigilant of its authenticity in being of service to others with a community of practice that lifts everyone to higher levels of morality and growth, focused towards achieving shared goals and personal aspiration."

Johns (2016) encourages us to create our own vision for leadership and to think beyond a list of attributes. From his perspective, leadership is a whole thing, requiring a whole statement. Given the complexity of leadership, writing a leadership vision is not an easy task. And, while language is limiting, it is essential to conveying and sharing ideas. Consider your own leadership ideas. What research and theoretical works on leadership influence you, your thinking, and your desired actions as a leader?

## ■ WHAT IS CARING LEADERSHIP?

I am now contemplating my own definition of caring leadership. According to Johns (2016), leadership can be viewed as movement from knowing your place to being in place as a transformational leader. Poignantly, Grissel Hernandez, a current doctoral student in the doctoral program in Caring Science at the University of Colorado, is studying this very topic for her dissertation. Facilitating her through a qualitative study of caring leadership will provide me with the opportunity to closely connect with my own being in place and vision as a leader. For now, my movement involves continuing to resonate with my own work and the work of others—reflecting on the words and actions that vibrate at a higher level, nurturing the human spirit of this work.

## PROFESSIONAL PRACTICES THAT EMERGE FROM CARING LEADERSHIP

There are professional practices of caring leaders that emerge from the Caritas Processes, caring literacy, self-exploration, and scholarship on leadership. The following serve as a general unfinished guide:

- Model the way—especially the courage to be vulnerable and authentically present with self and others
- Demonstrate the value of self-care through your own practices and encourage them among others
- Pause and reflect before engaging in interactions with others
- Create a caring/healing environment and openness to being in relationship with others
- Meet others where they are developmentally; thoughtfully consider the other person's frame of reference and point of view
- Actively listen and acknowledge positive and negative feelings
  - Respond authentically in a manner that encourages growth and preserves dignity and respect for all
  - Look for the best in others and hold them in high regard

## ■ CONCLUSION

I leave you with questions for reflection. Through mindful-awareness and reflective practice, these questions serve as a guide to deepen caring literacy and practices for caring leadership. Take time to contemplate these questions and listen with your heart as it connects you to your inner wisdom. Being still creates space to listen with the heart. I encourage you to consider your own vision for caring leadership. Together there is a collective power of loving hearts—loving hearts that lead to transforming health care, healing, and wholeness for all.

- What does it mean to be and become a caring leader?
- How do the Caritas Processes inform my thinking as a caring leader?
- What other higher vibratory words and actions are important to me as a caring leader?

- How do these words nurture the human spirit and soul of our work?
- How can I use the Caritas Processes and caring literacy as a guide for my own leadership development?
- What caring acts can I engage in today that model the way I intend to lead?
- How does reflective practice add depth to Caritas Literacy and practices of caring leadership?

## ■ REFERENCES

Anderson, R., & Adams, W. (2016). *Mastering leadership: An integrated framework for breakthrough performance and extraordinary results*. Hoboken, NJ: Wiley.

Brown, B. (2010). *The gifts of imperfection: Let go of who you think you're supposed to be and embrace who you are. Your guide to a wholehearted life*. Center City, MN: Hazelden.

Brown, B. (2012). *Daring greatly*. New York, NY: Gotham Books.

Dewey, J. (1933). *How we think: A restatement of the relation of reflective thinking to the educative process*. Boston, MA: D.C. Heath.

Gadamer, H. G. (1996). *The enigma of health. The art of healing in a scientific age* (J. Gaiger & N. Walkder, Trans.). Stanford, CA: Stanford University Press.

Horton-Deutsch, S. (2012). Learning through reflection and reflection on learning: Pedagogies in action. In G. Sherwood & S. Horton-Deutsch (Eds.), *Reflective practice: Transforming education and improving outcomes* (pp. 103–134). Indianapolis, IN: Sigma Theta Tau International.

Horton-Deutsch, S., Drew, B., & Beck-Coon, K. (2012). Mindful learners. In G. Sherwood & S. Horton-Deutsch (Eds.), *Reflective practice: Transforming education and improving outcomes*. Indianapolis, IN: Sigma Theta Tau International.

Horton-Deutsch, S., Pardue, K., Young, P. K., Morales, M. L., Halstead, J., & Pearsall, C. (2014). Becoming a nurse faculty leader: Taking risks by doing the right thing. *Nursing Outlook, 62*(2), 89–96.

Horton-Deutsch, S., & Sherwood, G. (2008). Reflection: An educational strategy to develop emotionally competent nurse leaders. *Journal of Nursing Management, 16*, 946–954.

Horton-Deutsch, S., Young, T., & Nelson, K. (2010). Becoming a nurse faculty leader: Facing challenges through reflecting, persevering, and relating in new ways. *Journal of Nursing Management, 18*, 487–493.

Johns, C. (2004). *Becoming a reflective practitioner* (2nd ed.). Carlton, Victoria, Australia: Blackwell.

Johns, C. (2006). *Engaging reflection in practice: A narrative approach*. Oxford, England: Blackwell.

Johns, C. (2016). *Mindful leadership. A guide for the health care professions*. London, England: Palgrave Macmillan.

Kabat-Zinn, J. (1990). *Full catastrophe living: Using the wisdom of your body and mind to face stress, pain, and illness*. New York, NY: Delta.

Kouzes, J., & Posner, B. (2003). *Academic administrators guide to exemplary leadership*. San Francisco, CA: Jossey-Bass.

Kouzes, J., & Posner, B. (2007). *The leadership challenge*. San Francisco, CA: Wiley.

Kouzes, J., & Posner, B. (2012). *The leadership challenge: How to make extraordinary things happen in organizations* (5th ed.). San Francisco, CA: The Leadership Challenge.

Lombard, K. (2011). *Nurses' experiences of the practice of the PeerSpirit circle model from a Gadamerian philosophical hermeneutic perspective* (Doctoral dissertation). Indiana University, Indianapolis, IN.

Lombard, K., & Horton-Deutsch, S. (2012). Creating space for reflection. In G. Sherwood & S. Horton-Deutsch (Eds.), *Reflective practice: Transforming education and improving outcomes*. Indianapolis, IN: Sigma Theta Tau International.

Pardue, K., Young, P., Horton-Deutsch, S., Pearsall, C., & Halstead, J. (n. d.). *Becoming a nurse faculty leader: Taking risks by being willing to fail*. (Submitted for publication.)

Pearsall, C., Pardue, K. T., Horton-Deustch, S., Young, P. K., Halstead, J., Nelson, K. A., . . . Zungolo, E. (2014). Becoming a nurse faculty leader: Doing your homework to minimize risk-taking. *Journal of Professional Nursing, 30*, 26–33.

Porter-O'Grady, T., & Malloch, K. (2007). *Quantum leadership: A resource for healthcare innovation* (2nd ed.). Burlington, MA: Jones & Bartlett.

Shapiro, S. L., Carlson, L. E., Astin, J. A., & Freedman, B. (2006). Mechanisms of mindfulness. *Journal of Clinical Psychology, 62*, 373–386.

Sitzman, K., & Watson, J. (2014). *Caring science, mindful practice: Implementing Watson's human caring theory.* New York, NY: Springer Publishing.

Stiles, K., Pardue, K., Young, P., & Morales, M. L. (2011). Becoming a nurse faculty leader: Practices of leading illuminated through advancing reform in nursing education. *Nursing Forum, 46*(2), 94–101.

Watson, J. (2005). *Caring science as sacred science.* Philadelphia, PA: F.A. Davis.

Watson, J. (2008). *Nursing: The philosophy and science of caring* (Rev. ed.). Boulder, CO: University Press of Colorado.

Wiklund Gustin, L., & Wagner, L. (2012). The butterfly effect of caring—clinical nursing teachers' understanding of self-compassion as a source to compassionate care. *Scandinavian Journal of Caring Sciences, 1*, 175–183. doi:10.111/j.1471-6712.202.01033.x

Young, P., Pardue, K., & Horton-Deutsch, S. (2015). Practices of reflective leaders. In G. Sherwood & S. Horton-Deutsch (Eds.), *Reflective organizations: On the frontlines of QSEN and reflective practice implementation* (pp. 49–67). Indianapolis, IN: Sigma Theta Tau International.

Young, P., Pearsall, C., Stiles, K., Nelson, K., & Horton-Deutsch, S. (2011). Becoming a nursing faculty leader. *Nursing Education Perspectives, 32*(4), 150–156.

# CHAPTER SEVEN

# The Co-Emergence of Caritas Nursing and Professional Nursing Practice in Peru

*Patrick A. Palmieri*

## CARITAS QUOTE

*Nursing can expand its existing role, continuing to make contributions to health care within the modern model by developing its foundational caring-healing and health strengths that have always been present on the margin. (Watson, 1999, p. 45)*

*Peruvian nursing, or* enfermería peruana, *has evolved as a vocation and somewhat apart from the international nursing community. The focus of many Latina scholars is to advance enfermería peruana from a vocation to a theoretically guided discipline with an established science. This chapter is the narrative, lived experience of a Peruvian American nurse who reflects on a 10-year journey to create space for the emergence of postmodern nursing in Peru. Dr. Palmieri comments on the state of the science and proposes a new future that is guided by Caring Science. To build South American* communitas, *he and others have worked to establish* Sociedad de Watson, *a Watson Caring Science Global Associate that links enfermería peruana to global Caritas, as described in other chapters in this book, that will build caring literacy through the translation of texts, the development of Caritas curricula for Latin American schools of nursing, and links to global Caring Science Scholars.*

## ■ OBJECTIVES

*The objectives of this chapter are to:*

- *Describe the state of the science of nursing practice in Peru*
- *Discuss how my work in performance improvement contributed to the success of advancing nursing as a discipline*
- *Advance the notion that Caritas nursing can develop nursing knowledge and informed practice*

Peruvian nursing, or *enfermería peruana*, is perceived as a vocation. Since the early 2000s, there has been increasing awareness of grand theories and a distinct disciplinary body of knowledge, but this is not yet widespread. Clinically, nursing's primary role is to carry out medical orders. The educational preparation consists of 5 years at the university; however, there are neither competency-based licensure examinations nor competency-based specialty certifications. The advanced practice role is currently being developed.

Nursing science in Peru is underdeveloped and often based on principles and methods borrowed from public health. In fact, most doctorally prepared nurses study public health rather than nursing theory and science. The situation in Peru is similar to Haynes, Boese, and Butcher's (2004) description of American nursing in the 1970s as evolving from a vocation to a profession grounded in a discrete and defined disciplinary knowledge. But this can be partially explained by the 1978 creation of the *Colegio de Enfermeros del Perú* (National Board of Nursing) and the 2002 law to create the Peruvian nurse practice act (Ministerio de Trabajo y Promoción del Empleo, 2002). In reality, enfermería peruana is young and immature but ready to grow with nurturing knowledge from the international nursing community.

Importantly, there is a proud nursing tradition in Peru, but this contributes to a partial disconnect of enfermería peruana from the global nursing community. For example, the nursing color in Peru is turquoise rather than purple (Rogerian) or white (sterile), the nursing day is celebrated August 30 instead of May 13 (Nightingale's birthday), and the Catholic Saint of Nursing is Saint Rosa of Lima, not Saint Camillus of Lellis (International Red Cross founder and official Vatican Saint of Nursing). There are no Sigma Theta Tau International (STTI) chapters in Peru, and there is no representative organization for enfermería peruana at the International Council of Nurses (2015). Overall, enfermería peruana is remarkably different than North American nursing and somewhat apart from the international nursing community.

This chapter describes my lived experience and professional reality as a Peruvian American nurse. These comments might seem ethnocentric, but I hope they may shed light on the current evolution of nursing in Peru. I speak about my lived experience as a relatively young male nurse, educated in the best American and

British universities, mentored by exceptional scholars in multiple disciplines, including nursing, management, education, and evidence-based health care, transitioning from an intellectually stimulating and beautiful Duke University campus to live and work in the exciting capitol of Lima, Peru. At the time and still true today, my relocation was motivated by my two loves in life: my new Peruvian wife, an accomplished economist and bank leader, and our nursing profession.

## ■ DEVELOPMENT OF GLOBAL NURSING KNOWLEDGE

The North American nursing tradition, with a remarkable history, evolved with the contributions of notable nursing scholars, including theorists, researchers, and practitioners. The discipline continues to gain strength and expand in visibility. From England, Florence Nightingale provided our initial call to action when she prepared women to care for the wounded and to comfort the dying soldiers during the Crimean War (Cook, 1913). Nightingale (1859) then emancipated our noble profession, stating:

> I use the word nursing for want of a better. It has been limited to signify little more than the administration of medicines and the application of poultices. It ought to signify the proper use of fresh air, light, warmth, cleanliness, quiet, and the proper selection and administration of diet—all at the least expense of vital power to the patient. (p. 2)

Continuing Nightingale's work, American nursing scholar Virginia Henderson (1966) further defined contemporary nursing for the International Council of Nursing, stating:

> The unique function of the nurse is to assist the individual, sick or well, in the performance of those activities contributing to health or its recovery (or to peaceful death) that he would perform unaided if he had the necessary strength, will or knowledge. And to do this in such a way as to help him gain independence as rapidly as possible. (Tomey & Alligood, 1998, p. 102)

Over the next 50 years, the nursing profession rapidly advanced. Importantly, the discipline emerged with the introduction of theories, matured with the synthesis of concepts, and the result is our theory-infused and informed practice (Meleis, 2007), the nursing praxis. This evolution emancipated nursing as a legitimate discipline; a carative health profession complementary to the curative medical partner (Watson, 2008).

Henderson introduced the Science of Unitary Human Beings (Rogers,1980), which was then advanced by Dr. Jean Watson to the Theory of Human Caring, to "explicate a distinct unitary view of human with a relational caring ontology and ethic that informs nursing as well as other sciences" (Watson & Smith, 2002, p. 461). The major elements contextualizing her theory to inform nursing practice include the carative factors, the transpersonal caring relationship, and the caring occasion/caring moment (Watson, 2001).

From Nightingale to Henderson, from Rogers to Watson, the North American nursing renaissance is expanding and informing the global nursing community. The renaissance is evidenced as Gallup (2015) again reported nursing as the most trusted profession, for the 14th consecutive year, noting, "With an 85 percent honesty and ethics rating—tying their high point—nurses have no serious competition atop Gallup ranking this year [2015]" (para. 1). I believe Dr. Watson is largely responsible for the American public's confidence in nursing. Dr. Watson (2012) believes nursing has evolved to advance positive social change from the individual to the global community:

> Nursing has consistently been affirmed by the public as ethical and worthy of public trust. Nursing's evolving science, theories, methods, and practices are expected to adhere to this public vision and hope for survival with integrity and purpose for this century and beyond. (p. 30)

For nursing to be defined in parsimonious worldview (Fawcett, 1993), we need a discrete and identifiable body of knowledge with theories and concepts constructed (Daly, 1997) to inform and guide nursing practice (Mitchell, 2002). Caring Science will inform this parsimonious worldview, including South America. Although nurses in South America have evolved as a discipline, they do not have enough knowledge to advance further (Mujica, 1982; Urra, 2009). My work is dedicated to my profession in Peru; to help my Peruvian colleagues achieve the public trust through advancing this worldview.

## TRANSITIONING CARING TO SOUTH AMERICA

Despite the North American nursing renaissance, countries in which the discipline of nursing is less developed continue with vocational nursing, or nursing practice not informed by a robust disciplinary knowledge and lacking theoretical-driven scientific inquiry. This is especially true in South America (Urra, 2009), where nursing struggles to emerge with a well-defined identity, literally fighting the suppressive sociomedico model. But, for the sake of their patients, Peruvian nurses may create their own roadmap, references from the North American caring–loving–healing tradition and knowledge. Advancing nursing from a vocation to a profession to a theoretically guided discipline with an established science is indeed the focus of many Latina nursing scholars. The Theory of Human Caring is a way for enfermería peruana "to see" (Watson, 2008), to know, to reflect, and to understand (Carper, 1978). This is where I will transition from the context into my personal story as I relocated to Peru to live and work nearly a decade ago, became a Peruvian citizen on July 4, 2012, and then met my mentor, Dr. Jean Watson.

In this chapter, I speak for the first time about my lived experience as a nurse working in the Andean region (Bolivia, Chile, and Peru) of Sudamérica. In particular, I focus on my new country, Peru. Cultural context is essential to explain how Caring Science and the Caritas Processes informed my leadership practices and provided me with the continued strength and courage to advance contemporary nursing knowledge in Peru. The word *Caritas* is especially meaningful to describe the way nurses bring caring, loving, and heart-centered care to patients and their families through their practice as well as accepting the same self-care into their personal life (Watson, 2009).

Enfermería peruana is poised to enter a new phase in development and could benefit from mentorship from academics, theorists, administrators, and advanced clinicians from other countries. With global nursing knowledge as the compass and the North American roadmap as a reference for the journey, the Caritas-informed nursing renaissance can be replicated in Peru. However, the discipline of nursing, as women's work, mimics the female role in society, which will be explained in the following section.

## PATERNALISTIC SOCIOMEDICAL CULTURE

The Peruvian health sector is especially challenging for nurses to navigate and disabling for nurses seeking to professionally advance as leaders. First and foremost, *enfermeras peruanas* (Peruvian nurses) are largely women working in a male-dominated and directed environment. The general Peruvian "machismo" culture extends with more purpose, a harsher reality, and nearly dictatorial style as traditionally male physicians control the health care sector. As a former health insurance executive responsible for the creation of the largest privately owned health system in Peru, I experienced working as a corporate and sector leader. My belief is that the Peruvian health sector is dominated not only by a "machismo" philosophy but also overlaps with a paternalistic sociomedical culture. But we need to heed the words of Nightingale (1859) as, "No man, not even a doctor, ever gives any other definition of what a nurse should be than this—devoted and obedient. This definition would do just as well for a porter. It might even do for a horse. It would not do for a policeman" (p. 200).

In this health sector culture, women are marginalized, including female patients, and often mistreated and sometimes harmed, emotionally and physically. Enfermeras peruanas are responsible for implementing physician orders and expected to comply without exception to directives issued by the "white jackets." These are the male physician hospital leaders who literally wear formal white blazers at work, a symbol of their power and sector status. With frequency, I observe nurses giving their chairs to physicians and I listen firsthand to accounts of sexual harassment and other injustices. Furthermore, I have witnessed instances of physical and verbal abuse against nurses in hospitals, including screaming, grabbing, and throwing objects. Finally, nurses work in unsafe and stressful environments. On the typical medical–surgical unit, the nurse-to-patient ratio ranges from 1:20 to 1:40; in the emergency department, the ratio is as high as 1:20. This reality begs the question whether or not enfermeras peruanas can engage in informed and reflective practice. The ratios, however, further evidence the lack of respect and concern for enfermería as an important Peruvian health profession.

## SITUATIONAL ASSESSMENT

Watson (1999) suggests nurses need to assess and critique their situations and see where or how they are in their environment, and then locate themselves within the framework or the emerging ideas in relation to their own paradigm of a caring professional nursing practice, including the relevant theories and philosophies. Furthermore, Watson (2001, p. 349) states,

> If one chooses to use the caring perspective as theory, model, philosophy, ethic or ethos for transforming self and practice, or self and system, the following questions may help: Is there congruence between (a) the values and major concepts and beliefs in the model and the given nurse, group, system, organization, curriculum, population needs, clinical administrative setting, or other entity that is considering interacting with the caring model to transform and/or improve practice? Are those interacting and engaging in the model interested in their own personal evolution? Are they committed to seeking authentic connections and caring-healing relationships with self and others? Are those involved "conscious" of their caring-caritas or non-caring consciousness and intentionally in a given moment and at an individual and system level? Are they interested and committed to expanding their caring consciousness and actions to self, other, environment, nature and wider universe? Are those working within the model interested in shifting their focus from a modern medical science-technocure orientation to a true caring-healing-loving model? (p. 350)

As such, enfermeras peruanas need to recognize their current practice environment, which negatively impacts their nursing work and their being. Furthermore, enfermeras peruanas can create the space to transform and improve their practice and their own personal development. Finally, through the Caritas, enfermeras peruanas can expand their own consciousness and shift the current paternalistic sociomedical orientation to embrace a nursing practice premised on caring–healing–loving relationships.

## ■ CONTEXT FOR CHANGE

Advancing enfermería peruana from vocation to profession requires the nursing practice to be informed by the disciplinary knowledge derived from Caring Science. When enfermeras peruanas receive international support and scholarly guidance, they can consciously shift their paradigm from the curative medical model to the carative nursing orientation, to practice caring–loving–healing. Through Caring Science, they can overcome mere compliance with the antiquated machismo sociomedical culture, displacing the medical ego, by engaging in reflective and Caritas-informed practice. As enfermeras peruanas increasingly understand the disciplinary knowledge offered by the Theory of Human Caring, they will embrace their new Caring Science paradigm and implement the Caritas into their daily self-care and patient care.

An assumption for intentional caring–loving–healing informed practice is the presence of a "safe space (sacred space) for people to seek their own wholeness of being and becoming, not only now but in the future, evolving toward wholeness, greater complexity and connectedness with the deep self, the soul and the higher self" (Watson, 1999, p. 102). When enfermeras peruanas establish their space, they can separate their identity from medicine by consciously and independently existing, developing, advancing, and achieving the wholeness in their caring–loving–healing practice, for self as well as others. When enfermeras peruanas establish their unique identity from medicine, their caring–loving–healing environment with a Caritas-infused practice, enfermería will become relevant to the health sector. Healing is an essential human attribute need which nurses offer to the public through their sacred practice.

Aware of the success with advancing hospital nursing through implementing nurse caring models grounded in Caring Science with Caritas-informed practices (Watson & Foster, 2003), from about 2007 to 2012 I led an ambitious agenda to clear a space for nursing with three strategies: (a) Develop nurse-led projects specific to quality improvement, patient safety, and risk management; (b) advance contemporary Caritas-informed practice by mentoring young and dynamic nursing leaders; and (c) exercise a new voice for nursing through public policy and political action. Then, in 2012, immediately after leaving the health system to focus on advancing enfermería peruana, my work sought to redefine nursing as a profession rather than a vocation with an established discipline defined by nursing knowledge instead of the legal constructs intended to restrain nursing. About a year after undertaking this work, I encountered resistance and experienced many failures. These experiences prompted extensive reflection and my return to reviewing the nursing literature and engaging in self-learning.

## HOW I CAME TO BEING WITH CARING SCIENCE

In early 2014, I was frustrated with the many barriers my Peruvian colleagues were facing as well as their reluctance to seek new ways of being and indecisiveness in embracing contemporary knowledge to inform their practice. At this point, I was stressed and not motivated to continue my work. In fact, I contemplated returning to the United States and possibly leaving nursing altogether. This was when I reached out to Dr. Jean Watson for help and, I hoped, some guidance. Really, I was desperate for an intervention, for help in learning more about Caring Science, and for encouragement to bring the practices of Caritas to my Peruvian nursing colleagues. But, at the time, the content of the intervention I sought was not fresh in my mind.

When I sent my first e-mail to Dr. Watson, I expected a response several weeks later; however, I was surprised with her immediate e-mail. This e-mail provided a sense of relief and new hope for me and my colleagues. After exchanging several e-mails, Dr. Watson invited me to attend her Research Intensive Proseminar 2 months later in Boulder, Colorado. Upon arriving at the Proseminar, I received an incredibly warm welcome and what I will call my first Caritas group therapy session. Most importantly, Dr. Watson helped me understand the world needs to change, to save humanity, and nursing is the profession responsible for stimulating this change through Caritas-informed practice. Leaving the Proseminar, I was resolute to become a human caring theorist and caring scientist. I realized I could lead a caring movement in Peru and throughout South America to create positive social change.

Officially in 2015, I became Dr. Watson's postdoctoral fellow, studying with and learning from the most influential nurse theorist since Florence Nightingale. And, my Caring Science studies and scholarly work continue with an incredible community of accomplished and enlightened faculty and scholars. Then, the real work began, understanding at the deepest level the philosophy underpinning Caring Science, learning the methodologies and methods, and understanding my praxis. My professional and personal lives are continuously informed by the Theory of Human Caring and guided by the principles set forth by the Caritas. Importantly, my actions and interactions remain mindful of the need to cultivate caring–loving–healing relationships and to practice loving-kindness (Watson, 2008).

## TRANSITIONING CARING SCIENCE FROM BOULDER TO LUCCA TO LIMA

While studying Caring Science and working with my Peruvian colleagues to begin our caring revolution in Lima, Peru, I began to achieve more successes than failures. In fact, I was inducted into the American Academy of Nursing as a fellow (FAAN) in October 2015. Prior to studying Caring Science, I was already a good scholar, something I did not fully appreciate. Thankfully, Drs. Alexia Green and Gayle Roux recognized my accomplishments and my ability to positively contribute to nursing in Peru, hence their sponsorship of my application. As I prepared my application I studied Caring Science, which inspired and motivated me through the process; the goal was to become a FAAN like my new mentor.

Ironically, perhaps coincidentally, I received the admission letter the week prior to traveling to Lucca, Italy, for the First Annual Caring Science Sacred Science Seminar. With my Caritas faculty and colleagues, I celebrated my news regarding my career transition. The seminar was notable for two reasons: First, I engaged in my first Caritas healing with art session, led by the creator, Dr. Mary Rockwood

Lane, who, in fact, contributed to this book. The small painting is framed and immediately visible on the right corner of my desk; a reminder of my past, the escape to the present, and the new Caritas path for the future. Then, following an incredible Puccini opera at a historic church, this book was literally conceived on a placemat as Drs. Lee, Watson, and I enjoyed a delicious pizza and shared stories about our journey to the Caring Science. In an important caring moment, we realized we are part of a developing global caring literacy, and our collective stories needed to be told.

## TRANSLATING CARING TO ACHIEVE OUTCOMES

By not only learning the Caritas Processes but living them, clear intentions and positive energy flooded my interpersonal field. Successes are constructed from loving caring intentions; however, I realize failures result when the ego escapes and dominates. Importantly, Caring Science guided the advancement of my practice to strengthen myself and to help me strengthen others; to support and expand our noble global profession; and to build our global communitas. To this end, the Asociación Peruana de Enfermería, or APE (Peruvian Nurses Association), was legally established in 2015 to inform and support enfermería peruana. The APE complements the National Board of Nursing by striving to advance nursing as a profession and discipline, guided and informed by Caring Science. But this professional organization was not sufficient to focus on advancing Caring Science. There needed to be an intentional focus to fill the space with caring–loving–healing energy.

Working with Dr. Watson and my colleagues, we realized there needed to be a direct link from South America to the Watson Caring Science Institute (WCSI). In April 2016, the *Sociedad de Watson* (Watson Society) was established within the APE to bring Caring Science to enfermería peruana, and to diffuse Caritas innovations throughout Sudamérica. These two organizations will continue our work to advance enfermería peruana as a discipline guided by the Theory of Human Caring, a nursing science defined by Caring Science, and a nursing practice informed by the Caritas. Through my early work, which is explicated in the next section, we cleared a space for nursing to begin practicing, teaching, researching, and leading as a Caritas-informed profession, complementary to our curative physician colleagues. Importantly, I worked to clear this space for enfermería peruana to embrace the Theory of Human Caring and to engage in Caritas-informed practice.

## ■ CLEARING THE SPACE AND BUILDING THE VOICE FOR PERUVIAN NURSING

Unlike North American nurses, enfermeras peruanas struggle to create a space for nursing, never mind the sacred space necessary for our Caritas-informed nursing practice. We have not been able to effectively advocate for our patients as our voice was weak and not focused with caring–loving–healing intentions. Drawing from my strength and preparation as a quality improvement and patient safety expert, I developed an international accreditation agenda, approved by my organization's leaders and endorsed by the board of directors, to develop the first nursing-led projects in a Peruvian health care facility. The rationale for implementing these nursing-led projects for enfermería peruana was to develop them as patient advocates through accepted medical concepts, quality improvement, and patient safety. This would be an opportunity to advance the profession and to establish the discipline defined by the Theory of Human Caring. My prime directive was clear—achieve an international accreditation with a nursing-led initiative within 3 years. With this directive, nursing would become an operationally relevant and recognized department within an emerging private health system.

Due to my positional power and professional reputation, my colleagues and I advanced nursing autonomy through results, proving better patient care through nursing-led quality improvement, patient safety, and risk management projects. The project began at the ambulatory oncology facility, then advanced to a private maternity hospital, and finally concluded at a small private hospital in the province of Peru. The initial space was established as each facility had a motivated visionary nursing leader supported by a chief executive officer (CEO) who trusted me in my belief that nurses could improve patient care and develop professional knowledge by implementing international standards guided by a theoretical framework.

## ■ THE LIVED EXPERIENCE OF CREATING A SPACE FOR NURSING

The quality improvement focused on implementing the international accreditation standards, guided by nursing and organizational science. The nurse leaders were intrigued with this seemingly strange theoretically guided framework. To the best of my ability, I led this project guided by Caring Science and Caritas-informed mentoring. This means, although not explicitly stated within the framework, I taught the Caritas factors and spoke the Caritas language as I mentored the nurse leaders, and even the CEOs, for each project.

Interestingly, my colleagues and mentees can now identify with this point, but I choose to quietly teach the Caritas to advance the carative processes to complement, rather than reject, the curative approach. And, I needed to be careful about how I described my goals and objectives to protect the project, and the nurses, from the machismo paternalistic forces that would prevent the space-clearing and voice-enabling agenda. In fact, my professional preparation as a nurse was neither discussed nor divulged by my non-nursing colleagues. But, focused on achieving results, I permitted others to temporarily shape my personal identity despite the uncomfortable feeling that I was hiding my nursing identity. The overall strategy led to many developments that I describe in the next section. However, I want to attribute the next exemplar outcome to my Caritas-informed leadership and Caritas-infused mentoring.

## NURSE-LED PROJECT EXEMPLAR

Although there is not sufficient space for reflecting on the projects, the operational results achieved by a nurse I continue to mentor were remarkable, providing a voice for nursing, allowing space for Caritas-informed practice to begin developing, and serving as an exemplar for others to replicate. At the start of the project, the self-evaluation demonstrated 27% compliance with all accreditation standards; incidentally, there were many problems with nursing turnover, physician satisfaction, adverse events, and financial results. After the project, the quality improvement data for each standard demonstrated an 86% compliance. Importantly, the standards deemed as "critical" rose to 100%. Furthermore, the operational balanced scorecard resulted in improvements in financial outcomes, a decreased number of adverse events with harm, and increased patient and physician satisfaction. The official accreditation evaluation resulted in no chapter deficiencies and a full 3-year accreditation.

The official accreditation is not the most significant project outcome, however. Through this quality improvement effort, where leaders fully engaged nurses and granted them permission to develop Caritas-informed practices, hospitals in developing countries can positively impact patient care. Importantly, these accreditation projects established nursing at each facility as the carative partner to our curative physician colleagues. Physicians began to recognize the power of caring–loving–healing relationships. When hospital leaders empower nurses to lead projects, such as quality improvement based on accreditation standards, and give them permission to develop independent nursing departments guided by nursing knowledge, remarkable transformations develop in patient care, resulting in increased patient and family, nurse, and physician satisfaction. In Peru, the importance of theoretically informed nursing practice has been underappreciated, often discounted, and generally not recognized as an essential quality improvement strategy.

Within 5 years from the start of the initial quality improvement/patient safety project, all three facilities achieved international accreditation and two have successfully been reaccredited. But the work extended past the nursing-led accreditation project as the space was cleared for nursing to evolve. With the reduced nurse-to-patient ratios in each of these facilities, caring can be practiced intentionally and nurses can have the Caritas consciousness, including the values and the motives, to create caring moments and to have an intentional consciousness of caring (Watson, 1988a, 1999). With more time, nurses can stop treating patients and begin engaging in caring–loving–healing nursing practices. The five core principles espoused by Dr. Watson (Watson, 2008, p. 34) can be embraced and incorporated into the soul of nursing practice. They are as follows:

1. Practice of loving-kindness and equanimity
2. Authentic presence: enabling deep belief of other (patient, colleague, family, etc.)
3. Cultivation of one's own spiritual practice toward wholeness of mind/body/ spirit—beyond ego

4. "Being" the caring–healing environment
5. Allowing miracles (openness to the unexpected and inexplicable life events)

Derived from the unitary human science of caring, the Theory of Human Caring is the nursing epistemology (Watson, 1988a, 1997). Later, the theory evolved into Human Caring Science (Watson, 2005, 2008, 2012) guided by 10 carative factors:

1. Formation of a Humanistic-altruistic system of values
2. Instillation of faith–hope
3. Cultivation of sensitivity to one's self and to others
4. Development of a helping–trusting, human caring relationship
5. Promotion and acceptance of the expression of positive and negative feelings
6. Systematic use of a creative problem-solving caring process
7. Promotion of transpersonal teaching–learning
8. Provision for a supportive, protective, and/or corrective mental, physical, societal, and spiritual environment
9. Assistance with gratification of human needs
10. Allowance for existential–phenomenological–spiritual forces (Watson, 1988b, p. 75)

Importantly, these elements of the theory are measured by the validated 10-item Caring Factor Survey. Here, the principle focus for each item is presented:

1. Practice loving kindness
2. Engage in decision making
3. Instill faith and hope in others
4. Teach and learn new things
5. Respect spiritual beliefs and practices
6. Provide holistic care
7. Establish helping and trusting relationships
8. Create a healing environment
9. Encourage the expression of feelings
10. Recognize and accept miracles (Adapted from DiNapoli, Nelson, Turkel, & Watson, 2010, p. 16).

However, in *Sudamérica* (South America), the 10 Caritas Processes are often called clinical Caritas, or *caritas clínicas* in Spanish (Favero, Joaquim-Meier, Ribeiro-Lacerda, de Azevedo-Mazza, & Canestraro-Kalinowski, 2009), reflecting the application of the theory to nursing practice.

These caritas clínicas represent the essential nursing praxis for Sudamérica; they define the *disciplina de enfermería peruana* (Peruvian nursing discipline) and advance the contemporary *practica de enfermería peruana* (Peruvian nursing practice). Enfermería peruana needs to join our global communitas and integrate the global Caritas praxis, or the "informed practice; practice that is empirically validated and informed by one's philosophical-ethical-theoretical orientation, but grounded in concrete actions and behaviors that can be empirically assessed and measured" (DiNapoli et al., 2010, p. 16). By defining the *disciplina de enfermería peruana* with the Theory of Human Caring, incorporating the Caritas into the *practica de enfermería peruana*, and studying nursing phenomena through *la ciencia de cuidado humano* (Human Caring Science), *enfermeras peruanas* can continue to expand their new space and strengthen their voice within the Peruvian health sector. The space is neither intended to compete with nor replace space occupied by medicine; however, the carative nursing space needs to coexist with curative medicine space to complement rather than compete.

Medicine is principally concerned with physical, largely mechanistic, curing, while nursing is concerned with holistic, or human, caring. In a Social Policy Statement (American Nurses Association, 1980), nursing was defined as "the diagnosis and treatment of human responses to actual or potential health problems." Unlike the physician focused on the disease, the nurse is concerned with the human response to it (Watson, 2005, 2008). As nurses and patients require caring relationships, healing environments, and a culture of caring, healing, and love, the "evolved integration and synthesis of Caring Science and Theory gives birth to authentic, spirit-filled, loving caring-healing practices that embrace all of humanity, offering a hopeful paradigm for this era" (Watson, 2010, p. 14).

With Caritas-informed practice, the nurse feels the "concern, regard, [and] respect one human being may have for another. Its roots lie in the maternal and paternal behavior of all higher living things, and it may be impaired or reinforced by environmental circumstances" (Sobel, 1969). In terms of physically curing, Hunt (1999) concluded, "The impersonal constructs of biomedical and social science are far removed from the inner life of fear, love and hope, an inner life which is, moreover, constantly in flux and, often, ambiguous" (p. 231). Because of the caring perspective, "the discipline of nursing arguably has the potential to develop unique knowledge of human health. It has this potential because nurses have a role within health care that gives them a privileged perspective on a range of issues" (Risjord, 2010, p. 77).

Importantly, Nightingale (1859) stressed the nurse–patient relationship is established to provide care by managing the internal and external environments in a manner consistent with the laws of nature. This is remarkably different from the work of physicians as Marcum (2009) opined, "rather than evidence-based practitioners, we should be striving to create epistemically virtuous physicians" (Upshur & Tracy, 2013, p. 1161). Because medicine is preoccupied with discovering cures in the positivist tradition, "it would make little sense to see medicine make a paradigm shift away from basic science" (Sehon & Stanley, 2003, p. 3). In medicine, the quantitative research, such as systematic reviews and randomized controlled trials, is considered the best evidence for practice (Straus, Ball, Balcombe, Sheldon, & McAlister, 2005), but this structural limitation has led medicine to be largely silent about integrating patient preferences and their values into an incompatible methodology. Consequently, contrasting movements such as patient-centered and person-centered care and values-based medicine have emerged as counterpoints to medicine to address this deficit (Miles & Mezzich, 2011), which is more complementary and reflective of carative-informed nursing practice.

## NEW SPACE FOR CARITAS-INFORMED PRACTICE

The private maternity hospital that achieved international accreditation engaged me to work with them to develop a new nursing reality. First, the hospital implemented a competency-based evaluation and salary scale premised on Benner's novice-to-expert theory (Benner, 1984). The nurse-to-patient ratios are guided by American nursing standards in all units, including neonatal nursery and intensive care units, perioperative services, and pre- and postpartum. Also, the hospital funded multiple 2-year nursing fellowships to develop nursing expert leaders in infection prevention and control, neonatal intensive care, and surgical services. Then, the hospital moved away from the traditional nursing structure, with a director of nursing reporting to the medical director, and a chief nursing officer (CNO) reporting directly to the CEO. The quality improvement director is a nurse, a position usually held by a physician. Next, the CEO developed a training and development area as well as a nurse relaxation room, which will emerge later this year as the *Espacio de Watson* (Watson Space). Finally, the hospital is funding nurse managers to seek MBAs and specialty nursing education. Each of these steps moves the organization along a pathway to prepare nurses for the final goal of changing the care delivery model. As such, I am actively engaged with the CEO and my bilingual mentee who was recently promoted to the CNO position in the initial preparations to develop a Caritas nursing model to support Caritas-informed nursing practice. When implemented, this will be the first theoretically guided nursing practice model implemented in Peru.

## POLITICAL ACTION FOR A NEW VOICE

In early 2015, nursing responded to the call for political action to change the machismo culture and paternalistic health sector when 13 nurses succeeded in becoming party candidates for the Peruvian Congress. The election resulted in two nurses earning seats in the Congress while another colleague fell slightly short of earning a seat. With two nurses in the Congress, there is a powerful voice to advocate for patients as well as the profession. In addition to the nurse seats in Congress, the nursing community rallied to force the Congress to approve a law to permit independent nursing practices to deliver health and wellness services.

## EDUCATION TO TEACH CARITAS

Private Peruvian schools of nursing are beginning to recognize Dr. Watson, like most prominent nursing scholars throughout the world, who was largely unknown in Peru until 2012. Similarly, there are no Sigma Theta Tau International (STTI) Honor Society for Nursing chapters in Peru; and there are only three in the entire

Latin America and Carribean region (2016). However, in 2015, the Peruvian Honor Society of Nursing began the process to achieve official STTI status, a process requiring 2 years (Sociedad de Enfermeria, 2016), and nurses in Bolivia and Chile are engaged in similar processes. After Dr. Watson presented at a university in Chiclayo, Peru. in 2015, there was excitement for learning the Theory of Human Caring and cultivating a Caritas-informed nursing practice. Dr. Watson continues to be invited to speak at Peruvian schools of nursing interested in establishing Caritas curriculums. In fact, Dr. Watson will speak twice in 2016 in Peru, including a 1-week engagement with the Colegio de Enfermeros del Perú (National Board of Nursing). The purpose of this visit is to help the National Board of Nursing understand how to construct a framework to infuse Caring Science into nursing education through the national accreditation process.

## ■ THE EVOLVING PERUVIAN COMMUNITAS

The Sociedad de Watson, a Watson Caring Science Global Associate, was established to connect Caritas nurses in pursuit of building a South American communitas. This interconnection between Caritas and communitas makes "explicit that we belong to a shared humanity and are connected with each other. In this way, we share our collective humanity across time and space and are bound together in the infinite universal field that holds the totality of life itself" (Watson, 2008).

A Watson Caring Science Global Associate (Global Associate) represents individuals, systems, projects, programs, and events from across the globe, endorsed and formally recognized by Dr. Watson and the WCSI. Each Global Associate is contributing to the development and advancement of Caring Science knowledge and practices in partnership with Dr. Watson/WCSI. The Global Associate designation identifies visionary leaders with Caritas-informed programs to address global caring needs of societies and communities. These leaders serve as inspired exemplars of Caritas-informed practice at this unique turning point for humanity. Global Associates seek to unite all health professionals under a shared commitment to embrace foundational and fundamental premises for sustaining human caring. The intended outcome is healing and health for all people around the globe (WCSI, 2016).

Through the increased presence of Dr. Watson in Peru and the mission of the Sociedad de Watson, the space for nursing continues to evolve as one devoted to Caritas-informed nursing practice. Importantly, the Sociedad de Watson is focused on bringing nursing leaders together through communitas. The next steps for the Sociedad de Watson include developing a pilot program called the Caritas Certified Curriculum for Latin American schools of nursing. Through this pilot certification program, we hope to stimulate additional interest and formative action to advance Caritas-informed nursing practice through a Caritas curriculum revolution. Finally, through the generosity of Dr. Kathleen Sitzman, the Sociedad de

Watson will be able to bring Spanish translations of education and development materials for Caring Science and mindful practice to Peruvian nursing and the evolving Sudamericana communitas. Upward and onward, we will move enfermería peruana, *vamos amigos*.

## ■ CONCLUSION

This chapter briefly described the traditional machismo and paternalistic environment where enfermeras peruanas practice; an environment not reported in the peer-reviewed literature. Then, the roadmap for the North American nursing renaissance was presented. Next, the exemplar project implemented to develop a space for nursing was described. And then, the curative versus carative epistemology was explained. Finally, the recent advancements were described and the relevance to the future plans was discussed. The Caritas revolution in nursing continues to advance from North America, to Europe, to Africa, to Asia, and now to South America through the WCSI scholars and postdoctoral fellows.

After nearly 10 years of work in Peru, the traditional practice environment is slowly being replaced with a new caring space for enfermería peruana. The result of Dr. Watson's frequent presence in Peru, physically and through social media, and my postdoctoral mentoring is a strengthened profession and development of a Caring Science-informed discipline. At this point, there is enlightened expansion as the vocation shifts to profession, informed by a carative epistemology. This is evident as three Peruvian universities have committed to establishing Caritas curriculums: Universidad Maria Auxilliar, Universidad Norbert Wiener, and Universidad Señor de Sipán

The work is making an impact. Last week, Dr. Watson and I traveled to Arequipa, Peru, to speak at the Human Caring Conference. And, Dr. Watson received two doctorate of honoris causa from prestigious Peruvian universities (Universidad Nacional de San Agustin and Universidad Católica de Santa María) for her contributions to global nursing and her current dedication to working with Peruvian nurses. And, I am quite proud of the honor bestowed upon me by the Alcade (Mayor) of Arequipa, *Vistante Distinguido* (Distinguished Visitor). The continued mentoring and guidance advances my knowledge and strengthens my plans: an evolution from expert practitioner to competent theorist, hopefully more.

With more time and tenacity, I will use the North American roadmap as my reference and the Caritas as my compass to mentor my own Caring Science mentees with the goal of experiencing an enfermería peruana renaissance within my lifetime. With Dr. Watson's help, this work is evolving and emerging in a different way. For example, Dr. Watson provides my talented bilingual mentee, Lic. Nataly Membrillo, the opportunity to serve as her translator for each trip to Peru. In order to translate for Dr. Watson, Lic. Membrillo has to study, understand, and internalize Caring Science. Through her visits, Dr. Watson graciously engages Nataly as a mentor, in her goal to become a Caring Science scholar. As I conclude this chapter, we should recognize Nightingale (the environment), Henderson (nursing definition), Rogers (unitary being), and then Watson (1996) provided us with the "critical, reflective practices that must be continuously questioned and critiqued in order to remain dynamic, flexible, and endlessly self-revising and emergent" (p. 143).

## ■ REFERENCES

American Nurses Association. (1980). *Nursing: A social policy statement.* Kansas City, MO: American Nurses Publishing.

Benner, P. (1984). *From novice to expert, excellence and power in clinical nursing practice.* Menlo Park, CA: Addison-Wesley.

Carper, B. (1978). Fundamental patterns of knowing in nursing. *Advances in Nursing Science, 1*(1), 13–24.

Cook, E. T. (1913). *The life of Florence Nightingale.* London, England: Macmillan. Retrieved from https://archive.org/details/lifeofflorenceni01cookuoft

Daly, J. (1997). What is nursing science? An international dialogue. *Nursing Science Quarterly, 10*(1), 120–122.

DiNapoli, P., Nelson, J., Turkel, M., & Watson, J. (2010). Measuring the Caritas processes: Caring factor survey. *International Journal for Human Caring, 14*(3), 15–20.

Favero, L., Joaquim-Meier, M., Ribeiro-Lacerda, M., de Azevedo-Mazza, V., & Canestraro-Kalinowski, L. (2009). Aplicación de la teoría del cuidado transpersonal de Jean Watson: Una década de producción brasileña. *Acta Paulista de Enfermagem, 22*(2), 213–218. doi:10.1590/S0103-21002009000200016

Fawcett, J. (1993). From a plethora of paradigms to parsimony in worldview. *Nursing Science Quarterly, 6*(2), 55–59.

Gallup. (2015, December 21). Americans' faith in honesty, ethics of police rebounds. Retrieved from http://www.gallup.com/poll/187874/americans-faith-honesty-ethics-police-rebounds.aspx?g_source=Social%20Issues&g_medium=newsfeed&g_campaign=tiles

Haynes, L., Boese, T., & Butcher, H. (2004). *Nursing in contemporary society: Issues, trends, and transition to practice.* Upper Saddle River, NJ: Pearson.

Henderson, V. (1966). *The nature of nursing: A definition and its implications for practice, research, and education.* New York, NY: Macmillan.

Hunt, S. M. (1999). The researcher's tale: A story of virtue lost and regained. In C. R. B. Joyce, H. M. McGee, & C. A. O'Boyle (Eds.), *Individual quality of life: Approaches to conceptualisation and assessment* (pp. 225–232). Amsterdam, Netherlands: Harwood Academic Publishers.

International Council of Nurses. (2015). Member list. Retrieved from http://www.icn.ch/members/members-list

Marcum, J. A. (2009). The epistemically virtuous clinician. *Theoretical Medicine and Bioethics, 30*(3), 249–265. doi:10.1007/s11017-009-9109-1

Meleis, A. I. (2007). *Theoretical nursing: Development and progress* (4th ed.). Philadelphia, PA: Lippincott Williams & Wilkins.

Miles, A., & Mezzich, J. E. (2011). The care of the patient and the soul of the clinic: Person-centered medicine as an emergent model of modern clinical practice. *International Journal of Person Centered Medicine, 1*(2), 207–222.

Ministerio de Trabajo y Promoción del Empleo. (2002, February 15). Ley Nº 27669: Ley del Trabajo de la Enfermera(o). Retrieved from http://www.mintra.gob.pe/contenidos/archivos/prodlab/legislacion/LEY_27669.pdf

Mitchell, G. (2002). Learning to practice the discipline of nursing. *Nursing Science Quarterly, 15*(3), 209–213.

Mujica, M. I. (1982). Aspectos polémicos sobre teorías y modelos de enfermería. *Revista Enfermería, 17*(74), 3–6.

Nightingale, F. (1859). *Notes on nursing: What it is and what it is not.* London, England: Harrison & Sons. Retrieved from https://archive.org/details/notesnursingwhat00nigh

Risjord, M. (2010). *Nursing knowledge: Science, practice, and philosophy.* West Sussex, England: Wiley-Blackwell.

Rogers, M. E. (1980). Nursing: A science of unitary man. In J. P. Riehl & C. Roy (Eds.), *Conceptual models for nursing practice* (2nd ed., pp. 329–337). New York, NY: Appleton-Century-Crofts.

Sehon, S. R., & Stanley, D. E. (2003). A philosophical analysis of the evidence-based medicine debate. *BMC Health Services Research, 3*(14), 1–10. doi:10.1186/1472-6963-3-14

Sigma Theta Tau International. (2016). *Latin American and Caribbean region.* Retrieved from http://www.nursingsociety.org/connect-engage/chapters/globalregions/latin-america-region

Sobel, D. E. (1969). Human caring. *American Journal of Nursing, 69*(12), 2612–2613.

Sociedad de Honor de Enfermería. (2016). *Introducción.* Retrieved from http://sociedadenfermeria.com

Straus, S. E., Ball, C., Balcombe, N., Sheldon, J., & McAlister, F.A. (2005). Teaching evidence-based medicine skills can change practice in a community hospital. *Journal of General Internal Medicine, 20*(4), 340–343. doi:10.1111/j.1525-1497.2005.04045.x

Tomey, A. M., & Alligood, M. R. (1998). *Nursing theorists and their work.* St. Louis, MO: Mosby.

Upshur, R. E. G., & Tracy, C. S. (2013). Is evidence-based medicine overrated in family medicine? *Canadian Family Physician, 59*(11), 1160–1161.

Urra, E. (2009). Avances de la ciencia de enfermería y su relación con la disciplina. *Ciencia y Enfermería, 15*(2), 9–18.

Watson, J. (1988a). New dimensions of human caring theory. *Nursing Science Quarterly, 1*(4), 175–181.

Watson, J. (1988b). *Nursing: Human science and human care. A theory of nursing.* New York, NY: National League for Nursing.

Watson, J. (1996). Watson's theory of transpersonal caring. In P. H. Walker & B. Neuman (Eds.), *Blueprint for use of nursing models: Education, research, practice, & administration* (pp. 141–184). NY: National League for Nursing.

Watson, J. (1997). The Theory of Human Caring: Retrospective and prospective. *Nursing Science Quarterly, 10*(1), 49–52.

Watson, J. (1999). *Postmodern nursing and beyond.* Edinburgh, Scotland: Churchill Livingstone/Harcourt-Brace.

Watson, J. (2001). Jean Watson: Theory of human caring. In M. E. Parker (Ed.), *Nursing theories and nursing practice* (pp. 343–354). Philadelphia, PA: F.A. Davis.

Watson, J. (2005). *Caring science as sacred science.* Philadelphia, PA: F.A. Davis.

Watson, J. (2008). *The philosophy and science of caring* (Rev. ed.). Boulder, CO: University Press of Colorado.

Watson, J. (2009). Caring science and human caring theory: Transforming personal and professional practices of nursing and health care. *Journal of Health and Human Services Administration, 31*(4), 466–482.

Watson, J. (2010). Caring science and the next decade of holistic healing: Transforming self and system from the inside out. *Beginnings, 30*(2), 14–16.

Watson, J. (2012). *Human caring science: A theory for nursing* (2nd ed.). Sudbury, MA: Jones & Bartlett.

Watson, J., & Foster, R. (2003). The Attending Nurse Caring Model: Integrating theory, evidence and advanced caring-healing therapeutics for transforming professional practice. *Journal of Clinical Nursing, 12*(3), 360–365.

Watson, J., & Smith, M. C. (2002). Caring science and the science of unitary human beings: A transtheoretical discourse for nursing knowledge development. *Journal of Advanced Nursing, 37*(5), 452–461. doi:10.1046/j.1365-2648.2002.02112.x

Watson Caring Science Institute. (2016). *Global associates.* Retrieved from https://www.watsoncaring science.org/global-caring-science

# CHAPTER EIGHT

# Creating Intentionality and Heart-Centered Leadership in the Hospital Setting

Jacqueline A. Somerville

### CARITAS QUOTE

*A transpersonal caring relationship is guided by an evolving Caritas Consciousness. It conveys a concern for the inner life world and subjective meaning of another. . . . Such an authentic spirit-to-spirit connection in a given moment transcends the personal ego level of professional control and opens the nurse's intelligent heart and head to what is really emerging and presenting itself in the now moment. (Watson, 2008, p. 79)*

*Nursing leaders who are guided by the Theory of Human Caring aim to ensure that caring remains the essence of nursing practice. Caritas-enlightened nursing leadership practices in this chapter are among some of the Caritas initiatives that have been implemented at Brigham and Women's Hospital in Boston, which is a National Caring Science Affiliate.*

### ■ OBJECTIVES

*The objectives of this chapter are to:*

- *Describe the rationale of bringing Caring Science to the academic medical center*

- *Describe the importance of caring literacy to advance nursing practice*
- *Describe strategies used in the implementation of caring-infused practice and leadership*

## ■ JOURNEY TO CARING SCIENCE AND CARITAS LITERACY

In 2011, I had the good fortune of becoming chief nursing officer (CNO) and senior vice president for patient care services at the Brigham and Women's Hospital (BWH). BWH is a 793-bed, Harvard-affiliated medical center, ranked sixth in the nation by *U.S. News & World Report* (2015). Situated in the Longwood medical district of Boston, Massachusetts, where research, practice, and education intersect, BWH employs nearly 3,000 extraordinary, world-class nurses.

Prior to my arriving at BWH, significant foundational work was accomplished by visionary nurses and leaders through appreciative inquiry, a process they aptly called, "finding the good" (Hickey & Kritek, 2012). This process guided nurses to reflect upon the good at BWH and to make sure the good remained a part of the culture. Through this process, nurses collaboratively developed the mission statement for the Department of Nursing: "Excellent care to patients and families, the best staff, in the safest environment." We later created a professional practice model, underpinned by inclusivity and caring intentions, that contains six domains:

1. Nurses as authentic leaders
2. Scholarship
3. Relationship-based care
4. Outcome-focused measures
5. Meaningful recognition
6. True collaboration

Relationship-based care was selected as our care delivery model, emphasizing care occurs within human relationships. The Department of Nursing created shared governance committees to encourage the collective nursing voice in decisions that impact them and their work. These six committees were:

1. Standards, Policies, and Procedures
2. Quality, Safety, and Care Improvement
3. Nursing Practice
4. Patient and Family Education
5. Informatics and Clinical Innovation
6. Nursing Research and Evidence-Based Practice

Professional practice models emerging from the early Magnet® work (McClure, Poulin, Sovie, & Wandelt, 1983) continue to evolve. Today, I see one of the top priorities in hospitals as developing and sustaining a human caring focus. This is particularly important in the large academic medical centers where the glory of technology may eclipse the person in the bed. In 2013, we invited Dr. Jean Watson to BWH as the Karsh visiting professor. I was impressed with Dr. Watson's message and how her words resonated with my nurse colleagues. I was convinced that our professional practice model would evolve into an even stronger model if it were theory-infused.

Although the early work to create professional practice environments was aimed at stemming the tide of an expanding nursing shortage, these professional practice environments are now an intentional and purposeful endeavor to support and advance professional nursing practice (Hickey & Kritek, 2012). The goal is for all nurses to be empowered and equipped to work to their fullest potential so that not only staff but also patients and families feel highly satisfied with the care experience. Resulting from the Magnet movement, nursing departments have established their own missions, visions, values statements, and professional practice models. More than 30 years since the original Magnet research was published, we need to ask the question, "Where should we be heading now?"

I believe great hospitals can check all the boxes of creating a professional practice environment: mission, vision, values statements, professional practice models, and shared governance models. However, we continue to strive for visible and measurable outcomes of nursing care. Yet, while checking these boxes is important, we need to return to our disciplinary foundation of caring and it may be hypothesized that quality metrics will follow. Therefore, our goal is to infuse human caring into all aspects of our professional nursing practice to advance a contemporary culture of care.

## ■ FOSTERING HEART-CENTERED LEADERSHIP

As the sixth-ranked hospital in the United States, BWH provides the finest nursing and medical care in the world. Our challenge is to retain caring as our disciplinary foundation because nursing can all too easily be swallowed up by the high technological agenda. Acutely aware of this challenge, some of our nurses use phrases such as, "humanizing the technology" or "taming technology" to remind us to complement care with the technology. Therefore, I highly value care and as a nursing department we set the goal to develop and sustain human caring practices.

This message was introduced by Dr. Watson when she initially visited our hospital. She implored nurses who were present in a standing-room-only audience to remember why they became nurses. Her loving and authentic question touched the hearts of nurses who reflected on why they entered the profession. This rekindled their passion for the discipline and renewed their commitment to caring. Nurses received Dr. Watson's message about the theory of caring and believed it to be applicable to their practices. I saw this acceptance as the strength of Caring Science—that it is not merely an academic theory. Instead, care is accessible to all and allows nurses to use it at the point of care.

Subsequently, our nurses began to think differently about their practice. Dr. Watson's message resonated with the nurses and moved many of them to tears. Her words did not confound nurses by using abstract theoretical language, but used clear words of caring. Nurses reflected, "How do I connect back to what brings meaning in my life, as a nurse?" "What brings me joy?" "What makes a difference to my patients and families?" "How do I stay focused not just on the beeps and alarms, but the person, through authentic presence, being able to listen, being able to read the field, and being able to integrate that which holds meaning to the patient?" These are all questions provoked by nurses reflecting about the relevance of caring in contemporary nursing practice.

When I saw the impact that Dr. Watson had on staff, it was an "a-ha" moment. Perioperative nurses, emergency nurses, procedural nurses, and nurses whom some might think would be less likely to move in the direction of theory-infused care were drawn back to why they became a nurse. Dr. Watson not only gave a presentation during her visit, she sat with nurses in different clinical areas and talked with them about their practice. The ability of the Theory of Human Caring to transcend to the point of nurses providing patient care is what makes it so accessible in a service-based environment.

The notion that we should honor every human being, and every time we touch a patient it should be considered a sacred act, is inspiring. Nurses are the environment of care through the intentions we bring to the bedside. Through our very presence at the bedside, patients either access healing energy, or they do not.

Dr. Watson's mid-range theory has become widely known through the 10 Caritas Processes. The Caritas reminds nurses in challenging moments to choose loving kindness and equanimity and to hold space for both the positive and the negative emotions. The Caritas Processes humanize every interaction with intention and remind nurses that being a nurse is an ontology—a choice about living and being in our world.

We have a covenant when we enter the room with the title "nurse" that calls us to the 10 Caritas Processes. I believe nurses, as the most trusted profession in the United States (Gallup, 2015), are the answer to healing our broken health system by practicing the Caritas. Every patient and family member I meet talks about wanting to be regarded as a whole, unique human being and cared for in the context of what holds meaning in his or her life. Nurses, therefore, in the community and at the bedside have opportunities to shift the whole environment to one filled with caring–healing energy.

As nurses, we witness daily profound human suffering—spiritual, physical, psychological—over the course of our careers. The only way to protect ourselves from cumulative grief is to shut off our hearts. If we were fully open to the experience without having a place to process the cumulative grief, we may go numb.

Dr. Watson teaches nurses to take care of themselves, to practice loving-kindness for themselves, so that they can be fully present for others. Reflecting on this notion of cumulative grief can be painful, at first. But, it is not about being a martyr. Practicing Caritas nursing, being fully present and open-hearted and engaged, causes you to receive the other in the transpersonal moment after which you are forever changed by the experience. One way we can foster this reflection is by asking, "Tell me about profound moments in your life that changed your practice forever." Next, I provide a paradigm moment in my own practice many years ago, as an example of a transpersonal moment that forever shaped me and my practice.

> *As I think about a paradigm moment in my career, it was while I was working on a vascular unit as a new graduate nurse. A gentleman had undergone successive amputations of his toes. He had severe ischemic pain but did not want to give up his leg at that point in his journey. We discharged him with medication to try to make his pain bearable. Sadly, he came back 3 weeks later, a shadow of himself. He finally made the decision to allow his leg to be amputated.*

> *An orderly came to put the patient on the stretcher for the operating room [OR]. The orderly came to me and said, "The patient wants to see you before he goes to the OR." I went to see the patient who said, "I just want to stand up one more time." I faced a dilemma because he had been premeditated. I was also a new grad and it was not acceptable to hold up the OR schedule. But, in those transpersonal caring moments, you know what's right to do. You just know it. All the other stuff goes out. You are so in the moment. You are so locked with that one human being that you cannot do otherwise, if you are a nurse. I helped him to his feet. He cried. I cried. But, if he had not done that, I am convinced that he would not have recovered. He made a decision. "I'm going to stand up one more time and then I am going to the OR in peace." His recovery was amazing. He was totally at peace with the decision. He was not in pain.*

Every nurse can identify the imprint of these transpersonal moments. They are immeasurable. To think that you had the honor to be in that moment with that person at that vulnerable moment in his or her life, that he or she trusted you, that you were doing the right thing by him or her, you are enriched by that forever. Transpersonal moments only take seconds but last a lifetime.

## ■ IMPLEMENTATION OF CARING THEORY-INFUSED PRACTICES

Theory-infused practice enriches our clinical environment by having nurses share a common language for what they do every day, their elegant practices that are often overlooked as routine or unexplored. Theory-infused practice is not an academic exercise but a life force that gives our work meaning and leads to the best possible outcomes for our patients and families. My goal is to see every patient/family/staff that enters our hospital feel welcomed and cared for. If you begin to live the Caritas Processes with your patients, families, peers, colleagues—when you are in the corridors, the cafeteria, or the community at large—it changes the environment forever. The 10 Caritas Processes also create a common language of caring for our hospital.

We have structural inequities in the health care system. At the point of care, however, there should be no inequities. Caritas leads us to care for all humanity with the same loving-kindness, trusting–caring relationships. Therefore, I see caring as a unifying force that binds us all in our mission.

To inspire others and leave bread crumbs along the path to Caritas, I will share the steps we have taken on our journey to become a National Caring Science Institute Affiliate. As previously mentioned, our Caritas journey began by hosting Dr. Watson in 2013 as the Karsh visiting professor. Estralita Karsh, wife of renowned photographer Yousef Karsh, has been a benefactress at BWH since 2001. Through her kind generosity, Mrs. Karsh not only provided the means of bringing Dr. Watson to BWH, but has also subsequently funded four leader/clinical nurse dyads to participate in the Caritas Coach Program. Our goal is to develop Caritas coaches as change agents in our culture. After mastering the Caritas Processes, coaches are expected to implement a Caritas project at their home institutions. I was privileged to attend the Caritas Coach Program in 2013 at the suggestion of Mrs. Karsh, who believed that the work would be expedited if the chief nurse were also a Caritas Coach. Touchstones is the name of my Caritas Coach project that has been sustained for over 2 years.

## ■ TOUCHSTONES

Nursing leaders often only convene for informational meetings and rarely find time for building communitas, defined by Watson as, "a shared humanity . . . connected with each other" (Watson, 2008, p. 93). In order to build communitas and promote a culture of caring, I decided to pilot a twice-weekly gathering of nursing leaders in a conscious and intentional way. Participation in Touchstones is completely voluntary and invitations are e-mailed to nursing leaders who have expressed interest.

As nurse leaders, we often practice in isolation, gathering only for meetings intended for information dissemination. Leaders influence the energy in the practice environment and our intentions shape the ability of the team to be wholeheartedly and fully present to patients and families. The Caritas environmental field model asserts that when one holds higher thought consciousness, the entire environmental field can be repatterned at a higher level.

Touchstones is a leadership practice in which approximately 30 nurse leaders gather at a brief, twice-weekly meeting to check in and foster collective consciousness through a poem, quote, music, or passage. Through voluntary participation, including the CNO and nurse executives, nurse directors, and program managers, the group is evolving toward a more intentional, reflective practice environment.

First, we check in with each other to determine the overall well-being of each other—not their units, problems, or crises—but as fellow human beings. Next, using the sound of our Watson singing bowl, we call the group together, whether in person or by phone, in mindful meditation, as taught by Dr. Watson (Watson, 2008). We focus on the rhythm of our breathing, spending 5 minutes to clear our minds toward an inner state of peace and stillness. At the close of the meditation, someone from the group offers an intention for the day, typically a quote, poem, or lyrics, after which members reflect and comment on its meaning to them. Collective consciousness for caring and healing has the potential to advance our common goal in the sacred clinical space and in our individual lives and community.

A focus group study was conducted to understand the value and experience of creating opportunities for nurse leaders to establish collective consciousness through Touchstones. Content analysis was used to analyze the data, resulting in five themes. First, leaders value Touchstones as leading to personal growth and self-awareness. Second, Touchstones resulted in communitas; participants stated that they felt good about gathering with like-minded people who have similar values and time to learn more about what each is struggling with, time to reflect together in a judgment-free zone. Third, Touchstones required moral courage by some nurse leaders who experienced resistance to the idea by peers. "Oh, this is the right work. There's no question in my mind that this is the right work and I believe that you can positively influence people and cultures." Fourth, Touchstones became the source of pride for the participants—pride in their CNO for her commitment to the practice. "It sets a standard, where you're in relationship with her. She sets a standard of authenticity and risk taking. . . . She's doing something that's cutting edge and it gives me permission to be creative." Fifth, participants were committed to sustaining Touchstones as it became an essential component of the leadership culture at the hospital. " . . . [H]olding authentic, heartfelt, positive thoughts such as loving-kindness, caring, healing, forgiveness, and so forth, vibrates at a higher level than having lower thoughts. . . . If one holds higher-thought consciousness, the entire field can be, and is being repatterned by the nurses' consciousness. . . . It requires personal-professional awakening, and an evolution toward a higher-deeper level of consciousness" (Watson, 2008, pp. 140–141).

Participant nurse leaders admitted that although some approached this new practice with some skepticism, it has become an important practice for them, not only at work, but at home, as well. Nurse leaders report using pausing and reflection-in-action prior to responding to the many demands, decisions, and problems of the day so that their responses were more intentional and heart-centered. In this way, they see themselves more heart-centered and better able to lead with loving-kindness. "We thus participate in creating reality, partially through our intentionality" (Watson, 1999, p. 12).

Other Caritas-infused practices are listed in the following text in order of implementation. They reflect a multipronged approach to Caritas. In addition to these milestones and Touchstones, described previously, there are seven additional Caritas Coach implementation projects that are ongoing. These are nurse-driven innovations, each exciting in their own right. One project, for example, is integrating a Caring Science approach to personhood into medical rounds. Nurses trained in Caritas Processes are reporting in rounds those things that are meaningful to the patient, not just laboratory values, imaging results, and vital signs. In fact, nurses are humanizing medical rounds by teaching the team about each spirit-filled person (Watson, 2008) and what really matters to him or her. Another example is infusing caring–healing practices in the primary care setting through loving-kindness, greater attention to that which is meaningful to patients and families, and greater loving-kindness and collaboration among staff. BWH nurses who are graduate students are also using Caring Science in their theses, capstones, and dissertations. Therefore, caring theory-infused practice, scholarship, and research has become the fabric of our being.

## ■ CREATING HEART-CENTERED LEADERSHIP

| | |
|---|---|
| 2013 | Dr. Jean Watson visits as Karsh visiting professor |
| 2013 | Chief nurse and a clinical nurse enroll in the Caritas Coach Program |
| 2014 | Caritas Processes are introduced at nursing leadership retreat |
| 2014 | Touchstones, a mindfulness exercise followed by a group intention, begins on Tuesdays and Fridays for all nursing leaders and continues to be sustained |
| 2014 | A nurse director and second clinical nurse enroll in the Caritas Coach Program |
| 2014 | Inaugural Lotus Award honors a clinical nurse |
| 2014 | Essence of Nursing Award recipient receives the Caring Science medallion |
| 2014 | Inaugural issue of *Heart & Science,* a monthly publication for members of Patient Care Services, is distributed |
| 2014 | Part 1: Caring Science and Heart Math Training for Nursing Leadership is offered |
| 2015 | Part 2: Caring Science and Heart Math Training for Nurse Leadership is offered |
| 2014–2015 | Advancement of a Caring, Healing, Healthy Environment is offered in the Connors Center for Women and Newborns |
| 2015 | Nurse director and a third clinical nurse enroll in Caritas Coach Program |
| 2015 | Director and program manager of integrative services become Caritas Heart Math coaches |

| 2015 | BWH Caring Survey distributed to 3,000 nurses |
| 2015 | Initial BWH Caring Survey results presented to nursing leadership |
| 2016 | BWH hosts the Massachusetts Regional Caring Science Consortium Conference |
| 2016 | Caritas Processes designated as the focus of six bimonthly nursing leadership seminars to build Caritas-enlightened leadership practices |
| 2016 | Nurse director and a fourth clinical nurse enroll in Caritas Coach Program, bringing the total to eight Caritas coaches |
| 2016 | Department of Nursing, BWH, hosts International Caritas Consortium in Boston |

## ■ CONCLUSION

"To become a National Caring Science Affiliate, an organization must demonstrate deep-rooted and sustainable commitment to integrating caring science within practices and policies, seeking to transform and broaden the notion of health and healing for its staff as well as the patients, families, and communities it serves" (Watson Caring Science Institute, n.d.). With this chapter, I hope to provide insight into the theory of caring and the theory-infused leadership practices that will transform and sustain a caring–healing environment for all.

## ■ REFERENCES

Gallup. (2015). Honesty/ethics in professions. Retrieved from http://www.gallup.com/poll/1654/honesty-ethics-professions.aspx

Hickey, M., & Kritek, P. B. (Eds.). (2012). *Change leadership in nursing: How change occurs in a complex hospital system.* New York, NY: Springer Publishing.

McClure, M. L., Poulin, M. A., Sovie, M. D., & Wandelt, M. A. (1983). *Magnet hospitals: Attraction and retention of professional nurses.* Kansas City, MO: American Nurses Association.

U.S. News and World Report. (2015, July 21). U.S. News & World Report releases 2015–2016 best hospitals. Retrieved from http://health.usnews.com/best-hospitals

Watson, J. (1999). *Postmodern nursing and beyond.* London, England: Churchill Livingstone.

Watson, J. (2008). *Nursing: The philosophy and science of caring* (Rev. ed.). Boulder, CO: University Press of Colorado.

Watson Caring Science Institute. (n.d.). National Caring Science affiliates. Retrieved from https://www.watsoncaringscience.org/national-wcsi-affiliates

# PART FOUR

# *Diverse Forms of Caritas Inquiry*

Research methods used to study Dr. Watson's Theory of Human Caring have been developed to ensure that inquiry into the phenomenon of interest is aligned with the moral–epistemological–ethical values of caring. During her doctoral study with Dr. Watson in the 1990s, Dr. Chantal Cara (Canada) expanded phenomenology so that human caring literacy forms the ontological basis for human inquiry in nursing. Her method, Relational Caring Inquiry (RCI), honors the relational human process between researcher and participant and is described by Dr. Cara and colleagues in this section. Next, a group of Italian nurses began what has become a 10-year collaboration with Dr. Watson, who mentored them in devising a method of inquiry of caring across health systems, which was congruent with caring and culturally acceptable to Italian nurses. Sandra Vacchi, Caritas Coach, describes the process that the Italian nurses undertook as they conducted the first Theory of Human Caring research in Italy. Dr. Gayle Casterline, a Caring Science Scholar and faculty in the Watson Caring Science Institute, who views nursing as a covenantal ethic of human service, uses heuristic inquiry to study spiritual health and spiritual care. Her travel and study in Ukraine resulted in a mixed methods study in which nurses offered stories of transpersonal caring moments as well as a heuristic study of prayer. Dr. Marcia Hills, longstanding faculty in the Watson Caring Science Institute and expert in Caring Science curriculum development, along with Dr. Simon Carroll (Canada), report on Collaborative Action Research and Evaluation (CARE), a relational inquiry that is well-aligned with the epistemology and ontology of Caring Science.

# CHAPTER NINE

# Relational Caring Inquiry: The Added Value of Caring Ontology in Nursing Research

*Chantal Cara, Louise O'Reilly, and Sylvain Brousseau*

## CARITAS QUOTE

*Developing knowledge of caring cannot be assumed; it is a philosophical-ethical-epistemic endeavor that requires on-going explication and development of theory, philosophy, and ethics, along with diverse methods of caring inquiry that inform caring-healing practices. (Watson & Smith, 2002, p. 456)*

*This chapter describes the journey involved in the creation of a research method, the Relational Caring Inquiry (RCI), developed by Dr. Cara, now a Distinguished Caring Science Scholar, Watson Caring Science Institute. This method was based on Husserlian phenomenology as well as a caring ontology. The elements of human caring literacy, especially Watson's work, informed this research method. The chapter also explores the shared venture by Drs. O'Reilly and Brousseau in utilizing this approach. In this way, the chapter exemplifies the creation and utilization of a theory-guided method of inquiry and shares our perspective regarding the added value of human caring ontology within research.*

## ■ OBJECTIVES

*The objectives of this chapter are to:*

- *Describe our personal journey within human caring literacy, specifically the creation of a research method and the shared venture of utilizing this approach within nursing research*

- *Demonstrate a theory-guided research methodology, based on caring ontology*

- *Discuss the meaning of being and becoming a caring researcher based on a human caring ontology.*

## ■ JOURNEY TO CARING SCIENCES AND CARITAS

In the following section, we present three personal stories that evoke the reasons beneath our choice to develop and use a phenomenological method, the Relational Caring Inquiry (RCI), to perform research within the discipline of nursing.

Dr. Cara was fortunate to be Dr. Jean Watson's doctoral student from 1991 to 1997 at the University of Colorado. Hence, being mentored by this great leader and inspired by her work over the years, she considered caring as the essence of nursing, not only within clinical practice but also fundamental to the research realm of nursing. Caring Science invited her to see what matters the most as being in relation with another human being and exploring the meaning of people's lived experiences. Of course, humanistic values have always played an important part in her life; however, Caring Science allowed Dr. Cara to put words on those inner beliefs, thus expending her consciousness toward her own moral ideal of being and becoming a caring nurse within her professional journey as a nurse researcher, teacher, and scholar. As early as 1985, Dr. Watson suggested the exploration of paradigm-transcending methods to study human caring and other phenomenon in nursing. Consequently, Dr. Watson's recommendation was illuminating in the development of a phenomenological method: the RCI (Cara, 1997, 1999). This research method was enlightened by the works of additional authors (Buber, 1970; Gadow, 1994; Husserl, 1970; Ray, 1991a, 1991b). Husserlian phenomenology primarily guides the data analysis and interpretation process, while Caring Science literacy provides a noteworthy ontology, since it assists the researcher in performing nursing research as a relational human process. Therefore, the ontology of caring allows this method to remain relational, dialogical, and transformative (Cara, 1997, 1999, 2002).

After several years of caring for patients and families, Dr. O'Reilly realized that the most significant nursing interventions were oriented on "being with" the person, a notion at the very heart of Watson's transpersonal caring relationship. To explore and better understand this relational understudied phenomenon, she achieved a doctorate at the Université de Montréal under Dr. Cara's supervision. She explored the meaning and contribution of the experience of "being with" the cared-for person, from the rehabilitation nurses' perspective (O'Reilly, 2007; O'Reilly & Cara, 2010). Later, she also studied the same phenomenon, but this time from the rehabilitation patients' perspective (O'Reilly, Cara, Avoine, & Brousseau, 2011). To study these eminently relational phenomena, Dr. O'Reilly selected the RCI, due to the caring ontological foundation, inviting us to see research as a relational process between the researcher and the research participants, and between the researcher and the *verbatim*. From Dr. O'Reilly's standpoint, a human caring ontology makes phenomenology more coherent and relevant to study nursing's phenomena of interest, such as those related to caring.

As for Dr. Brousseau, he observed for a decade that novice nurses refused to work in management as turnover was increasing. Inspired by Dr. Watson's work, he started a doctorate in nursing administration to study the meaning of nurse managers' quality of work life experience. Under Dr. Cara's supervision, Dr. Brousseau chose the RCI for its caring ontology, however, within a mixed methods research design, along with a quantitative methodology. With the RCI, he developed relational skills, essential in research, such as an authentic presence and continual respect for participants during interviews, allowing him to discover, without judgment, their lived experiences and co-create rich and meaningful narratives. Also, Dr. Brousseau acknowledged the added value of RCI within a mixed methods research design to provide meaningful solutions to problems experienced, for example, in nursing management (Brousseau, 2015; Brousseau, Cara, & Blais, 2016).

## ■ KEY ELEMENTS OF CARING SCIENCE AND CARITAS

In the following section, we review a selection of important Caring Science tenets acting as a keystone for the RCI's creation and utilization.

### RELEVANCE OF CREATING A NEW NURSING RESEARCH METHOD

In her works, Watson (1988, 2012) argued that:

> The methodologies that are relevant for studying my theory can be classified generally as qualitative-naturalistic-phenomenological field and interpretive, expressive methods of inquiry or a combined qualitative-quantitative inquiry versus a quantitative rationalistic method of inquiry as the exclusive method. . . . Nurses are encouraged to create new approaches that are appropriate for the phenomena under study. However, it is important to point out that these and other methods are in need of further development and practice. (2012, p. 94)

Dr. Watson's work was, therefore, inspirational to the development of a new method. Dr. Cara felt the need to expand phenomenology in order to enhance the research participants' contribution to the research findings. Informed by the Husserlian phenomenological process of analysis and interpretation, similarities exist between the RCI (Cara, 1997, 2002) and other phenomenological methods. Nevertheless, the caring ontology guided Dr. Cara to invite each participant for a second interview, allowing to reciprocate the story, analysis, and interpretation with the research participants, in order to seek, through a relational dialogue, a negotiation pertaining to the final meanings of their story. Also, it promotes the participants' contribution to provide new insights in regard to the phenomenon, going beyond a mere description of facts about people's experience, empowering them to share their ideas on how to improve problems or challenges regarding the phenomenon under study. Hence, the co-created meanings illustrate the contribution of both the researcher and the research participants through the relational dialogue (Cara, 1997, 2002).

## A CARING ONTOLOGY WITHIN NURSING RESEARCH

Hills and Watson (2011) stated the importance of an ontology of caring:

> Caring Science provides this deep underpinning for a scientific-philosophical-moral context from which to explore, describe, and research human caring-healing phenomena as integral to our humanity. As the disciplinary foundation for nursing, Caring Science clarifies for the profession, and the professional, the question of ontology, that is, what is our worldview of reality? What is the nature of Being and Becoming human in relation to the larger infinite universal field of life itself? (p. 13)

If caring ought to be the core of nursing (Hills & Watson, 2011; Watson, 1988, 1999, 2012), we trust that it should permeate the entire profession, including the research realm (Cara, 1997). In other words, caring should prevail in the nurse researcher's relationship with her research participants, not only in her relationship with her patients. Dr. Cara's research ontological perspective was enlightened by Caring Science literacy.

Underscoring an ontology of caring for nursing research, the research becomes a relational human process (Cara, 1997). This implies the researcher must "be with" the participants while sharing their meaning and experience regarding the phenomenon under study, honoring their voice throughout the research to remain "true" to their perceptions, beliefs, meanings, and stories pertaining to their lived experience. Hence, research participants are not considered mere subjects (or objects) to be scrutinized and fragmented; rather, the researcher aims to preserve their uniqueness, wholeness, and human dignity (Cara, 1997). In other words, we believe human caring literacy can provide an ontological basis for human inquiry in nursing in order to better relate "to" and "with" the world.

## INVITED CONTRIBUTION OF RESEARCH PARTICIPANTS TO KNOWLEDGE DEVELOPMENT

Watson (2005) proclaimed the following assumptions in regard to Caring Science:

> An ontological assumption of oneness, wholeness, unity, relatedness, and connectedness. An epistemological assumption that there are multiple ways of knowing, not only the physical sense data, but through tapping into our deep humanity our caring-healing relationship with self, Other, Nature, one's inner belief, accessing the infinity of life force of the universe, opening to something greater than oneself. . . . Caring science is grounded in a relational ontology of unity within the universe, which in turn informs the epistemology. (pp. 28–29)

Dr. Watson's assumptions are relevant to the RCI to focus on the relational caring process unfolding during the interview between the researcher and the participant. Therefore, human caring literacy leads the nurse researcher to consider the research participants as collaborators, contributors, or again, as experts in regard to the phenomenon under study, inviting a co-creation of meanings. According to O'Reilly (2007), the co-creation of meaning is largely induced by the authenticity within the dialogue being RCI's central element. In the absence of authentic dialogue, the participant's story will not be a co-creation associated with Buber's "I-Thou" relationship, but rather linked to Buber's "I-It" relationship (Cara, 1997; O'Reilly, 2007). In other words, without such dialogue, the researcher might not consider the research participants as contributors to knowledge development. Consequently, within the relational caring process, both the researcher and the participant have something to contribute to the phenomenon under study. Nevertheless, neither one holds the "absolute truth" (Cara, 1997). Moreover, Watson (2012) explained that a "caring moment" corresponds to a sacred space where two individuals can connect, interchange their perspectives, and come to a shared decision. In research, being informed by human caring ontology leads the researcher to create a "research caring moment." Hence, the unfolding within this "research caring moment" contributes to each person's transformation: a transformation of personal growth, insights, and consciousness, for both the researcher and the participants, as well as expanding knowledge in nursing, in regard to the phenomenon under study.

### ■ CARING THEORY IN OUR WORK

The following section first discusses the operationalization of the caring ontology deployed within the RCI (Figure 9.1). Also, the process of the RCI, which represents the circular phases of this method, is described (Figure 9.2).

## OPERATIONALIZATION OF THE CARING ONTOLOGY

For Husserl (1970), father of the phenomenological movement, phenomenology was a theory of knowledge, an "epistemology" rather than an "ontology." Thus, Husserl's work conveyed an epistemological perspective to nursing research rather than an ontological perspective (Cara, 1997, 2002). Therefore, a caring ontology can contribute, for the researcher, to enhance each participant's subjectivity and relation to the phenomenon through advocacy, openness, commitment, competence, authenticity, compassion, presence, and methodological rigor (Cara, 1997; see right part of Figure 9.1).

In addition, this ontology facilitates dialogue, mutuality, relationship, and negotiation between the researcher and the participant, hence inviting a co-creation of meanings (see middle section of Figure 9.1).

These aforementioned caring attributes (see right section of Figure 9.1) are essential to the RCI method. For instance, the role of *advocacy* is revealed through protecting research participants' human rights, respecting their confidentiality, and preserving the integrity of their stories. Watson (2014) also indicated that "moral justice framed within a sacred unitary worldview connects human-to-human caring with deep attention to both moral and social justice, including personal/professional action toward peace in our world" (p. 64). In the context of nursing research, however, we suppose the nurse researcher's advocacy would enhance human dignity at the participant level, thus protecting participants from being used as mere objects or providers of data.

As for the researcher's *openness*, it is imperative to encourage the participants' real stories and voices to be heard (Cara, 1997, 2002). Through Caritas Process #8, "Create a healing environment for the physical and spiritual self which respects human dignity," along with #5, "Allowing for expression of positive and negative feelings—authentically listening to another person's story," Watson (2007) emphasized the need for providing an environment filled with openness, trust, and support for people to allow them to feel comfortable in sharing their experiences with, in our case, the researcher. Openness makes it possible for the researcher to be entirely present and sensitive to the nuances in the participant's story as well as to ask clarifying questions, which could lead to a deeper understanding of the participant's experience (Cara, 1997, 2002).

For their parts, the researcher's *commitment*, along with the researcher's *competence* and *methodological rigor*, can be perceived as the cornerstones of quality research. Such attributes are exemplified within the method's philosophical foundation, the methodological process, as well as the validation and scientific rigor required in a study.

Dr. Cara (1997) also considered *authenticity* to be a relevant attribute for the researcher, as it remains an important attitude within human caring literacy, as the latter "seeks to create authentic, egalitarian, human-to-human relationships" (Hills & Watson, 2011, p. 17). Also, her fifth Caritas Process suggested that "authentically listening to another person's story" (Sitzman & Watson, 2014,

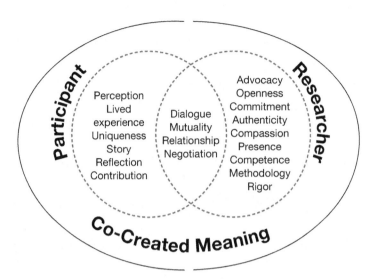

FIGURE 9.1   Participant–researcher's co-created meaning emerging from a caring ontology.
*Source:* Cara (2002).

p. 21) encourages her or his expression of feelings, in this case, the research participant. We believe that the greater the commitment of the researcher to establish
the relationship and the dialogue with the participants, the more the findings will
provide practical and experiential knowledge.

Dr. Cara (1997, 2002) considered *compassion* relevant while gathering the
participant's stories, as lived and experienced. Without compassion, the researcher
might not be open to the participants' stories. Indeed, as Watson (2003) stated,
"listening with compassion and an open heart, without interrupting" is essential
to grasp another person's story (p. 201). Watson explained that "Expressed compassion and caring is not only the word that is spoken or the eye that sees, leading
to action. The gaze itself is an expression . . . welcoming, receiving, affirming"
(2003, p. 200). In other words, the researcher's physical stance or attitude should
also be taken into account during the interview.

As for the last attribute, *presence*, Dr. Cara (1997) recommended being present to both the participant's story and the data throughout the entire research process. In her phenomenological method titled *Caring Inquiry*, Ray (1991a) also
emphasized the importance of the researcher's presence. Husserl's (1970) first phase
of his phenomenological reduction, named bracketing, also concerned the notion
of presence, as Watson (2012) explained:

> Husserl's ideal of phenomenology involved a different attitude: it
> involved *placing within brackets* the existential *historical aspect of experi-*
> *ence* and concentrating on the essence or the *ideal types* exemplified by
> the experiences that we either have or are able to conceive of ourselves
> as having. Phenomenology studies such essences and clarifies the vari-
> ous relationships between them. . . . Human phenomena (such as

caring, caring moments . . . ) are not object-like; they cannot be inspected or studied in the manner of objects. They have to do with the "how" rather than the "what." (p. 95)

Indeed, in order to be present to the participants and their stories, "bracketing" appears relevant to acknowledge both our own values and our own theoretical beliefs (Cara, 1997). Ultimately, we believe that the researcher's presence can help to share oneself, be authentic, and be open to the participants' stories. Indeed, Watson (2003) reminded us that "one's human presence never leaves one unaffected" (p. 200). In fact, according to Buber (1970), both persons must experience mutuality of presence, within an I–Thou relationship, in order for a genuine dialogue to take place:

> For inmost growth of the self is not accomplished, as people like to suppose today, in man's relation to himself, but in the relation between the one and the other, between men, that is, pre-eminently in the mutuality of making present—in the making present of another self and in the knowledge that one is made present in his own self by the other—together with the mutuality of acceptance, of affirmation and confrontation. (p. 70)

In brief, all these caring attributes assist the researcher ontologically to establish a relationship with each participant, in order to initiate a relational dialogue. Concretely, this relational dialogue takes shape in the participant's story, as well as the co-created meanings (or final findings; Cara, 1997; see also the middle section of Figure 9.1). More precisely, a relational caring ontology invites the researcher to understand the phenomenon with openness, consciousness, and humanness. It encourages both dialogue and mutuality between the researcher and the participants, hence sharing each individual's uniqueness, perspective, meaning, and creativity (see the left section of Figure 9.1). The co-created stories will become richer, reflecting participants' reality, while revealing the essential structures and essences of the phenomenon, thus contributing to new epistemology (Cara, 1997).

## THE PROCESS OF THE RCI

The following section outlines the process of the RCI (Cara, 1997, 1999, 2002; O'Reilly & Cara, 2014; Figure 9.2).

### Phase 1: Acknowledging the Researcher's Worldview

This phase, inspired from Husserl's (1970) notion of bracketing, corresponds to the acknowledgement of the researcher's values, context, and assumptions related to the phenomenon, in order to understand that one's background and underpinnings influence one's interpretations throughout the study (Cara, 1997; O'Reilly & Cara, 2014). We believe that such procedures promote listening to and honoring the participants' story. This is consistent with Dr. Watson's fifth Caritas Process (Sitzman & Watson, 2014).

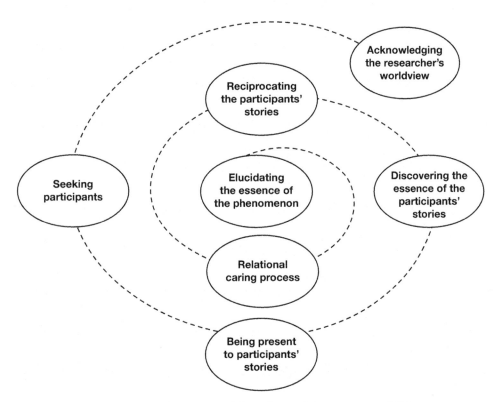

FIGURE 9.2   The process of the Relational Caring Inquiry (RCI).

## Phase 2: Seeking Participants

This step is concerned with advocacy and ethical responsibility as well as the selection of the participants. Besides the usual ethical procedures and assuring that confidentiality will be respected, each participant is asked to sign a written consent for both the audio-taped interviews (a minimum of two interviews will take place), along with its field notes (Cara, 1997). A resource should also be provided in case the participant would need to talk with someone after the interview (O'Reilly & Cara, 2014). As for the participants' selection, Lincoln and Guba (1985) recommended to remain open to a variation of exemplars in order to maximize the data collection. Benner (1994) suggested recruiting until the researcher reaches "redundancy."

## Phase 3: Being Present to Participants' Stories

This phase coincides with the interviewing moment. During the interview, the following open-ended question (first research question) is shared with each participant: *What is your meaning regarding* [the phenomenon under study]? The participants are asked to answer the question in the form of a story about a personal experience and to share it with the researcher: *Could you tell me a story about your personal experience regarding* [the phenomenon]? (Cara, 1997). As discussed previously, the researcher's presence, openness, and compassion are essential in this phase (Cara, 1997; O'Reilly & Cara, 2014) in order to carry out the interrogation as a "caring moment" (Cara, 2003; Cara & O'Reilly, 2008; Watson, 2012). Watson (2008) argued that it is essential to be present to, and supportive of, the expression of positive and negative feelings by allowing a story to emerge. Moreover, she specified that we must encourage narrative/storytelling as a way to freely express feelings, emotions, thoughts, ideas, beliefs, and values.

## Phase 4: Discovering the Essence of the Participants' Stories

Being inspired by Husserl's (1970) approach, this step relates to the analysis and interpretation of each participant's story in order to uncover its essence (Cara, 1997, 2002; O'Reilly & Cara, 2014). First, the researcher has to proceed with the transcription of each interview, then its transformation into a summarized story, which is followed by an analysis and interpretation aimed to seek the essence of the participants' lived experience (Cara, 1997; O'Reilly & Cara, 2014).

## Phase 5: Reciprocating the Participants' Stories

This phase endeavors to achieve mutuality between the researcher and each participant by helping them to clarify and expand their meaning pertaining to the phenomenon. In fact, being informed by a relational caring ontology, we believe that additional interviews encourage participants to validate and co-create findings. Thus, before the second meeting, a copy of the summarized story and its analysis are sent to each participant in order to provide any appropriate changes during the second interview (Cara, 1997; O'Reilly & Cara, 2014). Allowing them time to reflect can enhance a deeper understanding of their own perceptions. We believe that it is fundamental to share the analysis and interpretation process with the participant, in order to promote a relational dialogue (RCI's sixth phase) within the RCI (Cara, 1997).

## Phase 6: Relational Caring Process

This step targets the last interview and is characterized by the relational dialogue between the participants and the researcher (Cara, 1997; O'Reilly & Cara, 2014). Through this dialogue, the researcher seeks the participants' perceptions about the data analysis and interpretation (validation of the summarized story and its analysis) and solicits discussion and negotiation in order to foster a co-creation of meanings pertaining to the phenomenon for each participant (Cara, 1997; O'Reilly & Cara, 2014). During this phase, the researcher is also inviting the participant's advanced reflection or vision on how to improve or solve problems in regard to the phenomenon: *Could you share your perceptions on how we can promote* [the phenomenon]? Watson (2011) specified that "Caring accepts and holds safe space (sacred space) for people to seek their own wholeness of being and becoming, not only now but in the future, evolving towards wholeness, greater complexity and connectedness with the deep self, the soul and the higher self" (p. 103). In doing so, the researcher facilitates the participant's contribution to knowledge development (Cara, 1997). Indeed, Cara (1997) mentioned,

> One of the goals of the Relational Caring Inquiry is to be transformative. . . . During the relational caring process such transformation occurred through the dialogue and allowed for co-created meanings to develop. Empowering research participants to share their perspectives can facilitate their contribution of new knowledge on how to improve the phenomenon under study. (pp. 73–74)

Once again, an analysis and interpretation of the second interview's dialogue is realized by the researcher and sent to the participant for feedback. At the end of this phase, the researcher expresses her gratitude for the participant's contribution. Watson (2005) also acknowledged the importance of gratitude in a given moment, as it is "transforming in itself" (p. 117).

### Phase 7: Elucidating the Essence of the Phenomenon

This phase corresponds to the global analysis and interpretation of all participants' stories in order to elucidate the essence or essential structures of the phenomenon. To access the essence, Cara (1997) was inspired by Husserl's (1970) eidetic reduction, which corresponds to go beyond each particular individual's story toward the emergence of the universal meaning (or essential structures) of the phenomenon under study. To accomplish the eidetic reduction, free or imaginary variation is used to facilitate data agglomeration (Reeder, 1991). It consists of questioning the place of each element within a group of data to allow the emergence of the universal essence of the phenomenon under study as co-created meanings (Cara, 1997; O'Reilly & Cara, 2014; Figures 9.1 and 9.2).

## ■ CONCLUSION

This chapter highlighted the elements of human caring literacy, especially Watson's work, as fundamental to the development and utilization of a research method, the RCI (Cara, 1997, 1999, 2002; O'Reilly & Cara, 2014). We uphold the necessity for a reconciliation with the core of nursing, the ontology of caring, within research. If caring is a way of being, then should nurse researchers also be informed by this ontology? We need to value the caring presence and relationships, without embarrassment, while being a nurse researcher. It is essential to raise our awareness in broadening our view of nursing research, so as not to exclude the human caring literacy as a way of knowing, being, doing, and becoming a caring nurse researcher. After all, it is the nurses' right to care, even in research!

A relational caring ontology invites the researcher to understand the phenomenon under study with openness, consciousness, and humanness (Cara, 1997, 2002;

O'Reilly & Cara, 2014). It encourages both mutuality and relational dialogue between the researcher and the participants, thereby sharing each person's uniqueness, perspective, meaning, and creativity. The co-created stories will become deeper, reflecting the participants' reality, as perceived and lived (Cara, 1997). Without being considered exhaustive, the list of the aforementioned caring attributes is a starting point of what we consider significant to a caring ontology, as they are essential to the way of being and becoming a caring nurse researcher. Using the word *becoming* is paramount, since the RCI embraces a transformation for both the researcher and the participants. Such transformation emerges from the co-creation generated within the relational dialogue, encouraged by the relationship as well as the research caring moment. Indeed, one of the goals of the RCI is to be transformative (Cara, 1997, 1999, 2002; O'Reilly & Cara, 2014). Such perspective also appears to us as being coherent with a constructivist research paradigm (Creswell, 2013), since research participants can share their lived experience and co-create their meaning. Hence, the co-construction of the research findings, encouraged by the RCI's relational dialogue, seems consistent with the constructivism movement (Creswell, 2013). Truly, we believe that empowering research participants to share their perceptions and outlooks can enable their contribution to new knowledge on how to improve the phenomenon under study within nursing domains.

Finally, we also wanted to share our journey involved in the creation and utilization of this nursing research method. This journey has been both enriching and transformative for us, and is still in progress, using the RCI in mixed methods designs and in various domains of the discipline of nursing (Brousseau, 2015; Brousseau et al., 2016; Cara, 1997, 1999, 2002; Delmas, O'Reilly, Iglesias, Cara, & Burnier, 2016; O'Reilly, 2007; O'Reilly & Cara, 2010, 2014; O'Reilly et al., 2011). Hence, we are convinced that the RCI opens the path for the emergence of new epistemologies in nursing.

## THE ESSENCE OF OUR CHAPTER

*Nursing in this context may be defined as a human caring science of persons and human health-illness experiences that are mediated by professional, personal, scientific, aesthetic, and ethical human care connections and relationships. Such a view requires the nurse to be a scientist, scholar, and clinician but also a humanitarian and moral agent, wherein the nurse as a person is engaged as an active participant in the human caring process and relationships. (Watson, 2012, p. 66)*

## ■ DEDICATION

We would like to dedicate this chapter to the memory of Dr. Georgette Desjean, a professor, a nurse researcher, a mentor, and a friend. Dr. Desjean was a source of inspiration for introducing phenomenology at the Université de Montréal in the mid-1980s. A special thanks to all our research participants, who, over the years, have graciously shared their stories and co-created meanings with us.

## ■ REFERENCES

Benner, P. (1994). *Interpretive phenomenology: Embodiment, caring, and ethics in health and illness.* Thousand Oaks, CA: Sage.

Brousseau, S. (2015). *La signification expérientelle et les facteurs qui influencent la qualité de vie au travail des cadres gestionnaires infirmiers de premier niveau oeuvrant en établissement de santé [The experiential meaning and factors influencing quality of life at work of first line nurse managers working in health care]* (Unpublished doctoral dissertation). Université de Montréal, Montréal, QC, Canada.

Brousseau, S., Cara, C., & Blais, R. (2016). Experiential meaning of a decent quality of work life for nurse managers in a university hospital. *Journal of Hospital Administration, 5*(5), 41–52. doi:10.5430/jha.v5n5p41

Buber, M. (1970). *I and thou* (W. Kauffman, Trans.). New York, NY: Scribners.

Cara, C. M. (1997). *Managers' subjugation and empowerment of caring practices: A relational caring inquiry with staff nurses* (Unpublished doctoral dissertation). University of Colorado, Denver.

Cara, C. (1999). Relational caring inquiry: Nurses' perspective on how management can promote a caring practice. *International Journal for Human Caring, 3*(1), 22–29.

Cara, C. (2002). *Creating a caring environment in nursing research.* Paper presented at the Annual Conference of the International Association for Human Caring, Boston, MA.

Cara, C. (2003). A pragmatic view of Jean Watson's Caring Theory. *International Journal for Human Caring, 7*(3), 51–61.

Cara, C., & O'Reilly, L. (2008). S'approprier la théorie du Human Caring de Jean Watson par la pratique réflexive lors d'une situation clinique [Embracing Jean Watson's Theory of Human Caring through a reflective practice within a clinical situation]. *Recherche en Soins Infirmiers [Research in Nursing Care], 95,* 37–45.

Creswell, J. W. (2013). *Qualitative inquiry and research design: Choosing among five approaches* (3rd ed.). Los Angeles, CA: Sage.

Delmas, P., O'Reilly, L., Iglesias, K., Cara, C., & Burnier, M. (2016). Feasibility, acceptability and preliminary effects of an educational intervention to strengthen humanistic practice among haemodialysis nurses in the Canton of Vaud, Switzerland: A pilot study. *International Journal for Human Caring, 20*(1), 31–43.

Gadow, S. (1994). Whose body? Whose story? The question about narrative in women's health care. *Soundings: An Interdisciplinary Journal, 77*(3–4), 295–307.

Hills, M., & Watson, J. (2011). *Creating a caring science curriculum. An emancipatory pedagogy for nursing.* New York, NY: Springer Publishing.

Husserl, E. (1970). *The crisis of European sciences and transcendental phenomenology* (D. Carr, Trans.). Evanston, IL: Northwestern University Press. (Original work published 1954)

Lincoln, Y. S., & Guba, E. G. (1985). *Naturalistic inquiry.* Beverly Hill, CA: Sage.

O'Reilly, L. (2007). *La signification de l'expérience d'"être avec" la personne soignée et sa contribution à la réadaptation: la perception d'infirmières [The meaning of being with the cared for person and its contribution to rehabilitation: Nurses' perceptions]* (Unpublished doctoral dissertation). Université de Montréal, Montréal, QC, Canada.

O'Reilly, L., & Cara, C. (2010). "Être avec" la personne soignée en réadaptation: Une rencontre humaine profonde, thérapeutique et transformatrice ["Being with" the cared for person in rehabilitation: A deep, therapeutic and transformative human meeting]. *Recherche en soins infirmiers [Research in Nursing Care]*, *103*, 46–66.

O'Reilly, L., & Cara, C. (2014). La phénoménologie de Husserl [Husserl's phenomenology]. In M. Corbière & N. Larivière (Eds.), *Méthodes qualitatives, quantitatives et mixtes: Dans la recherche en sciences sociales, humaines et de la santé [Qualitative quantitative and mixed methods: In social, human and health sciences research]* (pp. 29–50). Québec City, QC, Canada: Presses de l'Université du Québec.

O'Reilly, L., Cara, C., Avoine, M. P., & Brousseau, S. (2011). Résilience: Pour voir autrement l'intervention en réadaptation [Resiliency: To see otherwise the intervention in rehabilitation]. *Revue Développement humain, handicap et changement social [Human Development, Handicap, and Social Change Journal]*, *19*(1), 111–116.

Ray, M. A. (1991a). Caring inquiry: The esthetic process in the way of compassion. In D. A. Gaut & M. M. Leininger (Eds.), *Caring: The compassionate healer* (pp. 181–189). New York, NY: National League for Nursing.

Ray, M. A. (1991b). Phenomenological method for nursing research. In *Summer Research Conference monograph: Nursing theory, research & practice* (pp. 163–172). Detroit, MI: Wayne State University.

Reeder, F. (1991). Conceptual foundations of science and key phenomenological concepts. In *Summer Research Conference monograph: Nursing theory, research & practice* (pp. 177–187). Detroit, MI: Wayne State University.

Sitzman, K., & Watson, J. (2014). *Caring science, mindful practice: Implementing Watson's Human Caring Theory*. New York, NY: Springer Publishing.

Watson, J. (1985). *Nursing: Human science and human care*. Norwalk, CT: Appleton-Century-Crofts.

Watson, J. (1988). *Nursing: Human science and human care* (2nd ed.). New York, NY: National League for Nursing.

Watson, J. (1999). *Postmodern nursing and beyond*. Edinburgh, Scotland: Churchill Livingstone.

Watson, J. (2003). Love and caring: Ethics of face and hand. *Nursing Administration Quarterly*, *27*(3), 197–202.

Watson, J. (2005). *Caring science as sacred science*. Philadelphia, PA: F.A. Davis.

Watson, J. (2007). 10 Caritas Processes™. Watson Caring Science Institute. Retrieved from https://www.watsoncaringscience.org/jean-bio/caring-science-theory/10-caritas-processes

Watson, J. (2008). *Nursing. The philosophy and science of caring* (Rev. ed.). Boulder, CO: University Press of Colorado.

Watson, J. (2011). *Postmodern nursing and beyond* (Rev. ed.). Edinburgh, Scotland: Churchill Livingstone.

Watson, J. (2012). *Human caring science. A theory of nursing*. Sudbury, MA: Jones & Bartlett.

Watson, J. (2014). Social/moral justice from a caring science cosmology. In P. N. Kagan, M. C. Smith, & P. L. Chinn (Eds.), *Philosophies and practices of emancipatory nursing: Social justice as praxis* (pp. 64–70). New York, NY: Routledge.

Watson, J., & Smith, M. C. (2002). Caring science and the science of unitary human beings: A transtheoretical discourse for nursing knowledge development. *Journal of Advanced Nursing, 37*(5), 452–461. doi:10.1046/j.1365-2648.2002.02112.x

# Collaborative Action Research and Evaluation: Relational Inquiry for Promoting Caring Science Literacy

*Marcia Hills and Simon Carroll*

## CARITAS QUOTE

*It is when we include caring and love in our science, we discover our caring-healing professions and disciplines are much more than a detached scientific endeavor, but a life-giving and life-receiving endeavor for humanity. (Watson, 2005, p. 3)*

*This chapter describes a research and evaluation inquiry process that is congruent with Caring Science and promotes Caritas Literacy. Collaborative Action Research and Evaluation (CARE) is a relational inquiry that does research and evaluation "with" people rather than "on," "to," or "about" them. This way of doing research is consistent with the ontology and epistemology of Caring Science and it provides a methodology and axiology that embrace human flourishing. Several exemplars are provided.*

## ◾ OBJECTIVES

*The objectives of this chapter are to:*

- *Articulate a research and evaluation approach (CARE) that is congruent with Caring Science and more particularly that advances Caritas Literacy*

- *Describe a research and evaluation inquiry process that shares and supports the ontology, epistemology, methodology, and axiology of Caring Science*

- *Expand Caring Science from "caring moments" between individuals to group dynamics that transform consciousness for collective wisdom*

- *Provide exemplars of projects in which CARE has been used to transform practices and systems to align with Caring Science*

## ■ JOURNEY TO CARING SCIENCE AND CARITAS LITERACY

This chapter explores the development of a research inquiry process that aligns and supports Caring Science and promotes Caring Science literacy. However, my (Hills) journey in Caring Science began long before I knew how to do research this way. I have spent 25 years using Watson's theory of caring in nursing education, culminating in a textbook, *Creating a Caring Science Curriculum: An Emancipatory Pedagogy for Nursing* (Hills & Watson, 2011). During this time, our School of Nursing at the University of Victoria became a Watson Collaborating Centre for Human Caring, focused mostly on nursing education (Bevis & Watson, 1989). Also, the Community Health Promotion Research Centre was established at the University of Victoria, of which I was the director. We had just received three federally funded research grants for projects using community-based research (CBR), a form of Collaborative Action Research and Evaluation (CARE). In addition, we were working in collaboration with a provincial funding agency to establish a training program to enable nonprofit community organizations to engage in this type of research. In 2008, I became a faculty associate and Caritas Coach at the Watson Caring Science Institute (WCSI). In 2010, Dr. Watson received an honorary degree from the University of Victoria for her dedication and commitment to our school's development. More recently, Dr. Watson had been pondering the idea of creating a nonaccredited doctorate in Caring Science, and I volunteered to assist her in its development. My coauthor on this chapter, Simon Carroll, joined me in 2003 at the Centre for Community Health Promotion Research at the University of Victoria. He and I continue to develop, write, and teach CBR and CARE. We have taught several multidisciplinary graduate courses and together have worked on several research projects, all of which use CBR or CARE. In 2013, Simon joined WCSI specifically to advise doctoral students, and to teach in the annual research doctoral proseminar. He and I are currently writing a book *Collaborative Action Research and Evaluation: A Catalyst for Health and Social Change* (Hills & Carroll, in press).

## ■ CARING SCIENCE AND CARE: SHARED VALUES, SHARED FOUNDATIONS

Caring Science has been described as "an evolving philosophical-ethical-epistemic field of study that is grounded in the discipline of nursing and informed by related fields" (Watson & Smith, 2002, p. 456). Like Dr. Watson, we believe that "caring" is the theoretical and philosophical disciplinary foundation for nursing (Watson, 1979, 2005).

Throughout her work, and particularly in her book *Caring Science as Sacred Science*, Dr. Watson (2005) argues that the traditional, separatist, orthodox approach to research is inadequate to address the philosophical, ontological, epistemological, and ethical perspectives that are inherent in Caring Science. Caring Science requires a different research paradigm, one that integrates a "critical self-reflexive consciousness with a deep experience of the sacred" (Reason, 1993, p. 282). As Reason explains, embracing this approach to research "would make a major contribution to what Maslow (1971) referred to as the 'further reaches' of human nature" (Reason, 1994b). Caring Science demands this approach to research. As Dr. Watson explains:

> As soon as one places caring within its science model or as soon as one locates the science model within the Caring Ontology (which is relational) science automatically grounds itself in it, and has the responsibility to attend to an ethical-moral-metaphysical stance. Caring forces us as individuals and professions to face our relation of infinite responsibility of belonging to other human beings as well as to a unitary field of all-our-relations. Such an orientation becomes non-dualistic, relational, and unified, wherein there is a connectedness of all. (Watson, 2008, p. 63)

As a Caring Science, nursing needs a different paradigm from which to conduct research. An orthodox, positivist paradigm is antithetical to the philosophical and theoretical foundations of Caring Science. When you introduce a "science of people," as we do in Caring Science, the ontology, epistemology, and methodology of orthodox research becomes inadequate to capture the human experience that is Caring Science. As Reason (1994b) explains:

> Orthodox research methods as part of their rationale, exclude human subjects from all forms of thinking and decision-making that generate, design, manage and draw conclusions from the research. Such exclusions treat the subjects as less than self-determining persons, alienates them from the inquiry process and from the knowledge that is its outcome and thus invalidates any claim that is its outcome and thus invalidates any claim the methods have to a science of persons. (Reason, 1994b, p. 346)

It is important to note that this is not a critique of orthodox research per se, but it is orthodox science's own declaration of what this type of research is trying to accomplish. From an orthodox research perspective, scientists want to take humans, who are the subjects of research, out of the equation. They are treated as "subjects without subjectivity," lacking any determinative agency; they are subjects *as* objects to be manipulated. Humans and their interpretations and purposes (practical, ethical, and spiritual) are treated as confounding variables that need to be "controlled." "A separatist model of science separates mind from body, eliminates any sense of spirit; such an orientation to science separates human from environment, from each other, from cosmos, which it seeks to control and manipulate as separate from one's own experience, one's own being" (Watson, 2005, p. 44).

However, from a Caring Science perspective, the opposite is true. The very aspect of being human that Caring Science seeks to understand, explain, and engage with is problematic from an orthodox science perspective. Because Caring Science is about people and our humanity, the nature of our relationship with the "subjects" of our research is a matter of paramount importance. We need to conduct research *in relationship* if we are to work truly in the spirit of Caring Science. We need a way of doing research "with" people, not "on," "to," or "about" them. It is this rationale that suggests a "participatory paradigm" of research is needed when doing Caring Science research.

CARE is congruent with the philosophical and theoretical foundations of Caring Science. CARE engages participants in an inquiry process that acknowledges the contributions that each participant makes to the creation of shared knowledge and wisdom; it is truly participatory and relational. Further, there is a consistency between the belief in a unitary field of consciousness (unity of mind–body–spirit–nature–universe in Watson [2005]) and the participatory worldview of CARE. As Heron and Reason (1997) explains:

> The participatory worldview allows us as human persons to know that we are part of the whole, rather than separated as mind over and against matter, or placed here in the relatively separate creation of a transcendent god. It allows us to join with fellow humans in collaborative forms of inquiry. It places us back in relation with the living world and we note that to be in relation means that we live with the rest of creation as relatives, with all the rights and obligations that implies. (Heron & Reason, 1997, p. 275)

Because of this rationale, we find that the most important and critical tenet of Caring Science is Caritas Process #4, "Developing and sustaining a helping trusting authentic caring relationship" (Watson, 2008, p. 31). This is the heart and science of nursing and CARE. The other Caritas Processes follow from this process. For example, you cannot form this type of relationship in Caring Science or CARE if you do not practice loving-kindness and equanimity for self and other—Caritas Process #1 (Watson, 2008, p. 31). Nor can you have this type of relationship if you are not authentically present (Caritas Process #2), or know how to use "self" and all ways of knowing (Caritas Process #6), or be able to teach from a coaching perspective (Caritas Process #7; Watson, 2008, p. 31).

In relation to Caritas Literacy, the CARE process is a structured platform that is congruent with the recognized need for a praxis of Caritas, where theoretical insight is embedded in, and unfolds from, the practice of Caritas, as a learning, caring, relationship-building mode of being. Just as Caritas Literacy asks us to become more fluent and confident in our caring practices, CARE as a research process asks us to take those same risks to the ego-bound self; to let go and engage with the other, in the moment of co-creation and knowledge building; into a deeper collaboration with others, as they and we bring our vulnerabilities into relation with each other to develop insight and effect meaningful, positive change in our relationships, our practices, our communities, and the global environment.

## ■ CARE

In this section, we outline the basic premises of CARE and establish it as an appropriate inquiry process that is congruent with Caring Science.

CARE is a particular form of participatory action research that is closely aligned with co-operative inquiry (Heron & Reason, 1997; Reason, 1988, 1994a). In fact, we use the methodology of co-operative inquiry within the CARE approach. Co-operative inquiry was developed in the late 1960s/early 1970s by John Heron, who determined "that only shared experience and shared reflection on it could yield a social science that did justice to the human condition" (Heron, 1996, p. 2). We prefer the terminology of collaboration rather than co-operation because co-operation does not capture the synergistic alliance that is integral to the success of this type of research approach. For us, the following definition best describes the caring collaborative relationship that we strive to create within the inquiry team:

> Collaboration is the creation of a synergistic alliance that honours and utilizes each person's contribution in order to create collective wisdom and collective action. Collaboration is not synonymous with co-operation, partnership, participation or compromise. Those words do not convey the fundamental importance of being in relationship or the depth of caring and commitment that is needed to create the kind of reciprocity that is collaboration. Collaborators are committed to, care about, and trust in each other. They recognize that, despite their differences, each has unique and valuable knowledge, perspectives and experiences to contribute to the collaboration. (Hills, 1991–1994; Hills & Carroll, 2016; Hills & Watson, 2011)

CARE is a planned and systematic process: Issues that are of interest to people, practitioners, or communities are formulated into researchable questions and plans are made for systematically collecting and analyzing data. "This formalized research process creates new knowledge upon which to base practice. It is the focus on the rigorous documentation of knowledge development that distinguishes

CARE from community development" (Hills & Mullett, 2000, p. 25). The following are the defining characteristics of CARE:

* *CARE is relevant to people and communities.* The research is grounded in the daily practices and activities of people, practitioners, or communities and results in decision making by those people or generates information that they can use to bring about change.
* *CARE requires participation.* The research is driven by a partnership between the community, the researchers, and other stakeholders, creating a synergistic alliance that maximizes the unique contributions of each participant.
* *CARE has a problem posing focus.* Designed to illuminate and seek solutions to practical problems, CARE focuses the research endeavor on the day-to-day activities and lives of community members, practitioners, and decision makers in order to make those activities more health promoting, humane, and caring.
* *CARE focuses on societal change.* The intent of CARE is that those involved will develop new ways of thinking, acting, behaving, and working by engaging in a collaborative research process.
* *CARE contributes to sustainability.* CARE is planned with sustainability in mind, often in the form of a new program that is developed or a new service that is delivered, and always through the enhancement of community or practitioner capacity to do future research and evaluation (Hills & Carroll, 2016; Hills & Mullett, 2000; Israel, Schulz, Parker, & Becker, 1998).

## A PARTICIPATORY PARADIGM

A paradigm is "a set of basic beliefs (or metaphysics) that deals with ultimates or first principles. It represents a worldview that defines, for its holder, the nature of the world, the individual's place in it, and the range of possible relationships to that world and its parts, as, for example, cosmologies and theologies do" (Guba & Lincoln, 1994, p. 105). Guba and Lincoln made a significant contribution in articulating four differing worldviews of research—positivist, postpositivist, critical, and constructivist—based on their ontological, epistemological, and methodological assumptions. Heron and Reason (1997) argue for a fifth worldview—a participatory paradigm. CARE is situated within this last paradigm and it embraces the ideology and methodology of co-operative inquiry created by Heron and Reason (1988, 1994a, 1994b, 1996, 1997) and Reason and Bradbury (2001).

A participatory paradigm rests on the belief that reality is an interplay between the given cosmos, a primordial reality, and the mind. The mind "creatively participates with [the cosmos] and can only know it in terms of its constructs, whether affective, imaginal, conceptual or practical" (Heron, 1996, p. 10). "Mind and the given cosmos are engaged in a creative dance, so that what emerges as reality is the fruit of an interaction of the given cosmos and the way the mind engages with it" (Heron & Reason, 1997, p. 279). As Skolimowski (1992) states, "we always partake of what we describe so our reality is a product of the dance between our individual and collective mind and 'what is there,' the amorphous primordial given-ness of the universe. This participative worldview is at the heart of the inquiry methodologies that emphasize participation as a core strategy" (p. 20). The participative perspective sees a world not of separate things, as a positivist view would have, nor as a socially reinforced construction of the human mind as held by the various relativist perspectives, but rather of relationships that we coauthor. The world we experience as "reality" is subjective–objective, a co-creation that involves the primal givenness of the cosmos and human experience, imagination and intuition, thinking and construing, and intentional action in the world (Heron, 1996). In participative knowing, knower and known are distinct, but not separate, parts of a unitary field of being, which is made up of relative independent entities, which unfolds through the process of coming to know and the action that derives from that knowing (Heron & Reason, 1997). In this view, "truth" is not a matter of static fact, but a quality of relationship (Abram, 1996, p. 264). This view is congruent with what Watson calls a unitary worldview that is "grounded in a relational ethical ontology of unity within the universe that informs the epistemology, methodology, pedagogy and praxis of caring in nursing and related fields" (Watson, 2008, p. 18).

## A RELATIONAL ONTOLOGY

Ontology refers to the form and nature of reality and what can be known about it (Guba & Lincoln, 1994). In contrast to orthodox research that utilizes quantitative methods in its claim to be value free (but which is more accurately described as valuing objectivity) and many qualitative approaches that value subjectivity, CARE endorses a relational stance, as does Caring Science.

A relational ontology means that there is "underneath our literate abstraction, a deeply participatory relation to things and to the earth, a felt reciprocity" (Abram, 1996, p. 124). As Heron and Reason (1997) explain, this encounter is transactional and interactive. "To touch, see, or hear something or someone does not tell us either about our self all on its own or about a being out there all on its own. It tells us about a being in a state of interrelation and co-presence with us. Our subjectivity feels the participation of what is there and is illuminated by it" (p. 279). So CARE is interested in investigating people's understandings and meanings as they experience them in the world.

At this ontological level, Caring Science and CARE share a fundamental phenomenological assumption that the world is constituted as relational; it assumes a subjective–objective duality, an always ready world for consciousness that spreads out before us and enlists us, throws us into its being. Before we analyze and separate, before we fall into a world of subject–object dualism (and mind–body, human–cosmos separation), we are part of one thriving, living cosmos, a unitary being that confronts us as our source and embeds within it a spiritual–ethical demand for caring. It is in the face of the other that we find an absolute obligation to be empathic, to recognize our connection, our oneness. CARE is a research process that takes on board these core philosophical assumptions, and builds an epistemic and methodological framework that follows logically from a deep relational ontology. We will have more to say about the specifics of this epistemological and methodological framework, but here it is important to stress that the rationale for a participatory paradigm is that we can only gain knowledge of our shared human world by recognizing the diversity of knowing; that the connection between seeing the other as worthy of our empathy and respect demands we also respect his or her knowledge, and his or her own ways of expressing that knowledge. These diverse ways of knowing constitute the core epistemic foundation for CARE; in the recognition of our fundamental unity, we have a commitment to respecting the contributions of diverse forms of knowledge.

## EXTENDED EPISTEMOLOGY

Epistemology refers to the nature of the relationship between the knower and what can be known. Guba and Lincoln (1994) claim that orthodox science, because of its belief in a "real" world that can be known, requires the knower to adopt a posture of objective detachment in order "to discover how things really are" (p. 108). There is a presumption that the knower and the known are separate and independent entities that do not influence one another. There is a search for the "truth"; for the facts in objective and quantifiable terms that hold empirical data in the highest esteem.

In contrast, CARE rests on an extended epistemology that endorses the primacy of practical knowing. In CARE, the knower participates in the known and that evidence is generated in at least four interdependent ways—experiential, presentational, propositional, and practical (Heron, 1996; Heron & Reason, 1997; Hills & Carroll, 2016).

### Experiential Knowing

Experiential knowing refers to direct encounters with persons, places, or things. "It is knowing through participatory, empathic resonance with a being, so that as the knower, I feel both attuned with it and distinct from it" (Heron & Reason, 1997, p. 281). Experiential knowing incorporates the participatory nature of perception as postulated by Husserl (1964) and Merleau-Ponty (1962). "Hardness and softness, roughness and smoothness, moonlight and sunlight, present themselves to us not as sensory contents but as certain kinds of symbiosis, certain ways the outside has of invading us and certain ways we have of meeting the invasion" (Merleau-Ponty, 1962, p. 317). Experiential knowing is "lived experience of the mutual co-determination of person and world" (Heron, 1996, p. 164).

## Presentational Knowing

Presentational knowing is grounded in experiential knowing and is the way we represent our experiences through spatiotemporal images such as drawing, writing, dance, art, or stories. "These forms symbolize both our felt attunement with the world and the primary meaning embedded in our enactment of its appearing" (Heron & Reason, 1997, p. 281). Watson illustrates the importance of these multiple ways of knowing when describing the intersection between science and the humanities. As she says, "The intersections between art and science help reveal the confines and contingencies of the invisible world so we 'see' that which is deeper, glimpsing the human spirit, the human soul, its beauty and loveliness, whatever its shape or form" (2008, p. 20).

## Empirical (or Propositional) Knowing

Empirical knowing is factual knowledge, knowing about something conceptually. This type of knowledge is usually expressed in terms of statements, facts, or theories. This way of knowing is of utmost importance in orthodox science inquiries and is relied on as the sole way to search for the "truth." In CARE, propositional knowing is seen as interdependent with the other three ways of knowing.

## Practical Knowing

Practical knowing has primacy in CARE. Practical knowing is knowing how to do something—it is knowledge in action. "Practical knowledge, knowing how, is the consummation, the fulfilment, of the knowledge quest" (Heron, 1996, p. 34). This form of knowing synthesizes our conceptualizations and experiences into action (practice).

Each form of knowing is to some degree autonomous and can be understood and can function on its own. However, of interest in this chapter is the interdependent nature of these four ways of knowing. Practical knowing, knowledge-in-action, is grounded in propositional, presentational, and experiential knowing (Heron, 1996). Intentional action or change is practical knowing. Consequently, change can be thought of as being based on evidence from all four ways of knowing. In CARE, as the inquiry group cycles through action and reflection, it builds theory (propositional knowing) from practice about what constitutes "good" practice. The inquiry team tests this theory in the real world of its practice and reflects on its experiences in relation to propositional knowing. The more congruent the four ways of knowing are, the more valid the evidence for practice and/or systems change. This participative epistemology articulates a way of knowing and acting that is both grounded in our experiential presence in the world and honors the human capacity of sense-making and intentional action (Reason, 1998, p. 12).

Caring Science, Caritas, and Caring Literacy all acknowledge and rely upon this respect for diversity and the authentic contribution of each being in its own unique unfolding, as we build up our knowledge of the world as part of a collaborative endeavor. Whether it be between nurse and patient, or any other set of relationships, all are imbricated in a complex multiplicity of knowing, taking in all aspects of our self-expression, as we explore the given cosmos together. It is in this way that both Caring Science and CARE share a perspective that sees authentic collaboration as both a principled ethical stance, as well as the foundation for the search for understanding/knowing.

Before turning to a discussion of axiology, it is pertinent to further consider this relationship of theory to practice as it is critical in understanding evidence-informed practice for practitioners and communities.

## PRAXIS—THE RELATIONSHIP OF THEORY TO PRACTICE IN CARE

Theory is often talked about as if it belongs in the world of the academy; some form of abstraction that is separate from our day-to-day lives. Simply defined, theory is an explanation of phenomena (Hills & Watson, 2011). It is our contention that theory is implicit in all human action and is critical in developing evidence for practice. "Only theory can give us access to the unexpected questions and ways of changing situations from within" (Schratz & Walker, 1995, p. 107). It is the relationship of theory to practice that is key in CARE. As Lewin (1947) declared many years ago, "there is nothing so practical as a good theory and the best place to find a good theory is by investigating interesting problems in everyday life" (p. 149).

In contrast to orthodox science, CARE does not see theory as something that is known and that "informs" practice. As van Manen (1990) suggests, "practice (or life) comes first and theory comes later as a result of reflection" (p. 15). In CARE, it is the cycling through the iterations of action and reflection in which experiential knowing and propositional knowing are considered in relation to practical knowing that creates praxis and generates evidence for future practice. This process grounds practice in theory rather than applying theory to practice.

This notion of praxis is a fundamental concept in Freire's work (Friere, 1972; Shor & Friere, 1987) and is fundamental to creating evidence-informed practice and communities. Praxis does not involve a linear relationship between theory and practice wherein the former determines the latter; rather, it is a reflexive relationship in which both action and reflection build on one another. "The act of knowing involves a dialectical movement which goes from action to reflection and from reflection to new action" (Freire, 1972, p. 31). Through critical dialogue, people become "masters of their thinking by discussing the thinking and views of the world explicitly or implicitly manifest in their own suggestions and those of their comrades" (p. 95). Praxis, therefore, is constituted by both a theoretical and an experience component and is mediated by dialogue. As Wallerstein (1988) explains, "the goal of group dialogue is critical thinking by posing problems in such a way as to have participants uncover root causes of their place in society—the socio-economic, political cultural, and historical contexts of people's lives" (p. 382). It is through this emancipatory dialogue that people are liberated to act in ways that enhance society. Conceptualizing the relationship between theory and practice this way reorients our thinking about research from searching for understanding and explanation to ethical action toward societal good (Hills & Mullett, 2000).

## AXIOLOGY

In addition to considering the three defining characteristics of a research paradigm suggested by Guba and Lincoln—ontology, epistemology, and methodology—Heron and Reason argue that an inquiry paradigm also must consider a fourth factor—axiology.

Axiology deals with the nature of value and captures the value question of: "What is intrinsically worthwhile?" The fourth defining characteristic of a research paradigm, axiology, puts in issue "values of being, about what human states are to be valued simply because of what they are" (Heron & Reason, 1997, p. 287). The participatory paradigm addresses this axiological question in terms of human flourishing. Human flourishing is viewed as a "process of social participation in which there is a mutually enabling balance, within and between people, of autonomy, co-operation and hierarchy. It is conceived as interdependent with the flourishing of the planet ecosystem" (Heron, 1996, p. 11). Human flourishing is valued as intrinsically worthwhile and participatory decision making is seen as a means to an end "which enables people to be involved in the making of decisions, in every social context, which affect their flourishing in any way" (Heron, 1996, p. 11).

In this way, human flourishing is tied to practical knowing, knowing how to choose, how to be, and how to practice in ways that are not only personally fulfilling but that also enhance and transform the human condition. This is similar to Freire's (1972) notion of conscientization. As he explains, "Even when you individually feel yourself most free, if this is not a social feeling, if you are not able to use your freedom to help others to be free by transforming the totality of society, then you are only exercising an individualistic attitude towards empowerment and freedom" (p. 109). This valuing of human flourishing reconnects individuals to human communities and recognizes the "truth" in our actions and practices. It means that in CARE what is of interest is more than the usual research outcome. As Freire (1972) so eloquently states, "The starting point . . . must be the present, existential, concrete situation, reflecting the aspirations of the people . . . .[We] must pose this . . . to the people as a problem which challenges them and requires a response—not just at an intellectual level, but at a level of action" (p. 75). As Reason (2006) goes on to explain, "The focus on practical purposes draws attention to the moral dimension of action research—that it is inquiry in the pursuit of worthwhile purposes, for the flourishing of persons, communities, and the ecology of which we are all a part" (p. 188). This conceptualization expands Caring Science from an individual focus to a group understanding with the intention to create collective wisdom and societal change.

The utility of the outcome of CARE is judged based on the difference it makes to transform the health and well-being of the people, practitioners, decision makers, and communities.

## ■ A METHODOLOGY AND METHODS FOR CBR

The terms *methodology* and *methods* are often confused. For our purposes, we define *methodology* as a conceptual framework for doing research that is grounded in theory. *Methods* are the techniques and procedures we use for collecting data.

## METHODOLOGY

One methodology that is particularly well suited to CARE is co-operative inquiry (Heron, 1996; Reason, 1994a, 1994b). Co-operative inquiry is a participatory action methodology that does research "with" people, not "on," "to," or "about" them. This methodology engages people in a transformative process of change by cycling through several iterations of action and reflection. Co-operative inquiry consists of a series of logical steps including identifying the issues/questions to be researched, developing an explicit model/framework for practice, putting the model into practice and recording what happens, and reflecting on the experience and making sense out of the whole venture (Reason, 1988). It is the explicit focus on theory and model development that creates opportunities to advance Caritas Literacy and practice, by asking questions like "What would it look like if we practiced from a Caring Science perspective?" or "What would it look like if we practiced by implementing the 10 Caritas Processes in our work?" This is followed by developing an explicit model/framework for practicing this way and then trying it out in our day-to-day practice and collecting data systematically so that we can change/transform our practice and our literacy in Caring Science. Then, evidence about what constitutes "best practice" is generated by people examining their practices in practice and reflecting on these practices and literacy.

## METHODS

As stated earlier and as should now be obvious, CBR is not and cannot be method driven. The methods used to collect information about people and the human condition derive from and are contained by the principles of CARE, the research question, and the methodology (including a theoretical framework).

In Caring Science and CARE, the research questions are almost always focused on wanting to know something about people or the human condition. At the heart of the critique about orthodox inquiry is that the methods are neither adequate nor appropriate for the study of persons because persons are, to a significant degree, self-determining. To provide evidence for practice that involves people, those people themselves must be involved in deciding what the appropriate methods are for collecting evidence and how the evidence can be interpreted. "To generate knowledge about persons without their full participation in deciding how to generate it, is to misrepresent their personhood and to abuse by neglect their capacity for autonomous intentionally. It is fundamentally unethical" (Heron, 1996, p. 21).

Gadamer (1975) argued that a preoccupation with objective methods or techniques is antithetical to the spirit of human science research scholarship. "The research questions themselves are the important starting point, not the methods as such" (van Manen, 1990, p. 1). An interesting dialectic exists between the researcher and the research question: How one chooses to frame the question influences how one chooses to investigate it. It seems reasonable to expect a certain harmony between the researcher (as a person), the research question, and, subsequently, the methodology and methods.

In CARE, whichever method is chosen, it needs to accommodate the notion of full participation of those involved. As a result, qualitative methods such as interviewing, journal writing, taped interactions, critical incidents, narrative accounts, and focus groups are likely to be used. In our experience, this criterion of using appropriate methods has challenged Caring Science practitioners and researchers to develop new and innovative strategies to access people's experiences and understanding. This way of thinking about research and the resultant methods that are used provide convincing evidence upon which to practice and to be in the world.

## ■ EXEMPLARS OF CARE

For the past several years, we have engaged in a number of funded research projects that have each used this research approach to build capacity in not-for-profit NGOs, practitioners, and decision and policy makers to make research more democratic; to deal with social justice; to promote health; and to change health systems toward inclusive and people-centered caring relational practice. All of these research projects are consistent with the tenets of Caring Science. We began with a mandate from a provincial funding organization, the British Columbia Health Research Foundation (BCHRF), to develop capacity in CBR (a form of CARE) with community NGOs, which challenged the academy as the intellectual "owner of research knowledge" and agendas. "Within a participative worldview, inquiry is not the province of specialist researchers, but rather becomes a way of life which integrates action with reflection, practice with learning" (Reason, 1993, p. 275). This work was coupled with federal funding to systematically develop a program of CBR within the academy (Hills & Mullett, 1999–2003). With the restructuring of the Canadian Institutes of Health Research (CIHR) funding came the opportunity to use this democratic inclusive person-centered research approach to change health care systems (Hills, 2003; Hills & Mullett, 2005a, 2005b; Hills, Mullett, & Carroll, 2007) and include people who had typically been excluded from decision making in the research process—people who had research done to them without their participation. From these later two projects, we began to appreciate the importance of having policy and decision makers in the same room with practitioners. Their ability to solve issues collaboratively was powerful. We started to reconceptualize CBR as CARE in order to recognize the contribution of all members of the inquiry team.

Recently, we have been engaged in two research projects that use this research approach with policy makers to promote health through partnerships and cross-sector collaborations. This work has developed out of a movement within health promotion focused initially on *Promoting Health Through Intersectoral Action* (Geneau, Hills, & Mitic, 2011–2013), and has more recently been approached from the perspective of *Health in All Policies* (Hills et al., 2014–2016). We have worked with our local provincial government (British Columbia), along with the Government of Canada, using a CARE approach to develop evidence concerning how to more effectively plan, implement, and sustain intersectoral policy for better health outcomes. Although there are significant differences in the rhythm and nature of the CARE process when working with policy makers, our experience has shown that the fundamental principles of CARE and Caring Science still apply, no matter what type of stakeholders we are engaging. Everyone wants to have his or her knowledge respected and integrated into the research process in a way that truly catalyzes a participatory engagement and produces practical and effective change.

Watson (2005) herself confirms this congruence between CARE and Caring Science when critiquing Reason's (1993) work as she says, "The notion of a living, sacred cosmos, within Reason's view, can inform our notions of inquiry so we can develop a new kind of sacred science" (p. 25).

In conclusion, Reason (1988) reminds us:

> [I]t is possible to inquire systematically and rigorously into a field of human action, and do justice to its wholeness without distorting or fragmenting it; it is possible to link inquiry and action in fruitful and illuminating ways; it is possible to co-opt bust practitioners into committed inquiry into their own professional and personal processes; it is possible for co-researchers to descend into the confusion of chaos and order that is real life without the protective clothing of questionnaires, experimental designs, and other forms of defensive armour, and to emerge with worthwhile understandings. (p. 125)

## ■ REFERENCES

Abram, D. (1996). *The spell of the sensations.* New York, NY: Pantheon.

Bevis, E. O., & Watson, J. (1989). *Toward a caring curriculum: A new pedagogy for nursing.* New York, NY: National League of Nursing.

Freire, P. (1972). *Pedagogy of the oppressed*. London, England: Penguin Books.

Gadamer, H. (1975). *Truth and method*. New York, NY: Seabury.

Geneau, R., Hills, M., & Mitic, W. (2011–2013). *Promoting health through intersectoral action* (formerly The Case of ActNowBC in British Columbia). Ottawa, ON, Canada: Canadian Institutes of Health Research (CIHR).

Guba, E., & Lincoln, Y. (1994). Competing paradigms in qualitative research. In N. Denzin & Y. Lincoln (Eds.), *Handbook on qualitative research* (pp. 105–118). Thousand Oaks, CA: Sage.

Heron, J. (1996). *Co-operative inquiry: Research into the human condition*. London, England: Sage.

Heron, J., & Reason, P. (1997). A participatory inquiry paradigm. *Qualitative Inquiry, 3*(3), 274–294.

Hills, M. (1991–1994). *Collaborative Nursing Program of British Columbia. Annual Reports*. Submitted to Curriculum and Professional Development Centre. Victoria, British Columbia: University of Victoria.

Hills, M. (2003, June). *Using participatory action research to encourage reflective, multi-disciplinary, evidence-based practice in primary health care*. Paper presented at the Ninth International Reflective Practice Conference: Mindful Inquiry, Cambridge, England.

Hills, M., & Carroll, S. (2016). Evaluating a community health program: Collaborative action evaluation. In A. R. Vollman, E. Anderson, E. T., & J. McFarlane, *Canadian community as partner: Theory & multidisciplinary practice* (4th ed.). Philadelphia, PA: Wolters Kluwer.

Hills, M., & Carroll, S. (in press). *Collaborative action research and evaluation: A catalyst for health and social change*. New York, NY: Springer Publishing.

Hills, M., & Mullett, J. (1999–2003). *Promoting evolution of disciplines through multi-disciplinary collaborative community-based research. Development of a research program for collaboration and participation in community research*. Social Sciences and Humanities Research Council (SSHRC), Research Development Initiative (RDI). Victoria, British Columbia: University of Victoria.

Hills, M., & Mullett, J. (2000). *Community-based research and evaluation: Collaborative action for health and social change*. Centre for Community Health Promotion Research. Victoria, British Columbia: University of Victoria.

Hills, M., & Mullett, J. (2005a). Primary health care: A preferred health service delivery option for women. *Health Care for Women International, 26*(4), 325–399.

Hills, M., & Mullett, J. (2005b). Community-based research: A catalyst for transforming primary health care rhetoric into practice. *Primary Health Care Research and Development, 6*(4), 279–290.

Hills, M., Mullett, J., & Carroll, S. (2007). Community-based participatory research: Transforming multi-disciplinary practice in primary health care. *Revista Panamericana de Salud Publica [Pan American Journal of Public Health], 21*(2/3), 125–135.

Hills, M., Paton, A., Desjardins, S., Fortune, K., Harrington, M., Sieben, M., . . . Mitic, W. (2014–2016). *Health in all policies: A realist synthesis of context-sensitive policy mechanisms for sustainable implementation*. Ottawa, ON, Canada: Canadian Institutes of Health Research.

Hills, M., & Watson, J. (2011). *Creating a Caring Science curriculum: An emancipatory pedagogy for nursing*. New York, NY: Springer Publishing.

Husserl, E. (1964). *The idea of phenomenology*. The Hague, Netherlands: Martinus Nijhoff.

Israel, B. A., Schulz, A. J., Parker, E. A., & Becker, A. B. (1998). Review of community-based research: Assessing partnership approaches to improve public health. *Annual Review of Public Health, 19*(1), 173–202.

Lewin, K. (1947). Feedback problems of social diagnosis in action. *Human Relations, 1*, 147–153.

Maslow, A. H. (1971). *The farther reaches of human nature*. New York, NY: Penguin.

Merleau-Ponty, M. (1962). *Phenomenology of perception*. London, England: Routledge & Kegan Paul.

Reason, P. (Ed.). (1988). *Human inquiry in action*. London, England: Sage.

Reason, P. (1993). Reflections on sacred practice and sacred science. *Journal of Management Inquiry, 2*(3), 273–283.

Reason, P. (Ed). (1994a). *Participation in human inquiry*. London, England: Sage.

Reason, P. (1994b). Three approaches to participative inquiry. In N. Denzin & Y. Lincoln (Eds.), *Handbook of qualitative research* (pp. 324–339). Thousand Oaks, CA: Sage.

Reason, P. (1998). Political, epistemological, ecological and spiritual dimensions of participation. *Studies in Cultures, Organizations and Societies, 4*, 147–167.

Reason, P. (2006). Choices and quality in action research practice. *Journal of Management Inquiry, 15*(2), 187–203.

Reason, P., & Bradbury, H. (2001). Inquiry and participation in search of a world worthy of human aspiration. In P. Reason & H. Bradbury (Eds.), *Handbook of action research: Participative inquiry and practice* (pp. 1–14). London, England: Sage.

Schratz, M., & Walker, R. (1995). *Research as social change*. London, England: Routledge.

Shor, I., & Freire, P. (1987). *Pedagogy for liberation: Dialogues on transforming education*. South Hadley, MA: Begin & Garvey.

Skolimowski, H. (1992). *Living philosophy: Eco-philosophy as a tree of life*. London, England: Arkana.

van Manen, M. (1990). *Researching lived experience: Human science for an action sensitive pedagogy*. London, ON, Canada: Althouse Press.

Wallerstein, N. (1988). Empowerment education: Freire's ideas adapted to health education. *Health Education Quarterly, 15*(4), 379–394.

Watson, J. (1979). *The philosophy and science of caring*. Boston, MA: Little Brown.

Watson, J. (2005). *Caring science as sacred science*. Philadelphia, PA: F.A. Davis.

Watson, J. (2008). *The philosophy and science of caring* (Rev. ed.). Boulder, CO: University Press of Colorado.

Watson, J., & Smith, M. (2002). Caring science and the science of unitary human beings: A transtheoretical discourse for nursing knowledge development. *Journal of Advanced Nursing, 37*(5), 452–461.

CHAPTER ELEVEN

# Spirituality and Nursing: United States and Ukraine

Gayle L. Casterline

---

### CARITAS QUOTE

*We open our hearts and minds to seek a deeper, more intimate relationship with that which is greater than self, the Divine. We open to prayer, to humility, to asking for what we need from the larger universe through acts of faith and hope. (Watson, 2008, p. 194)*

---

*This chapter offers a window into my life as a nurse and a woman of faith. It offers a view of my Caritas journey and how I have learned to be whole and in-the-moment within the Caring Science paradigm. Caritas living informs my roles as nurse/leader/mentor and wife/mother/citizen. I have focused on my exploration of spirituality and health, as well as some insights about spirituality and nursing in Ukraine.*

## ▇ OBJECTIVES

*The objectives of this chapter are to:*

- *Illuminate the harmony and joy in my life through theoretical thinking and being*
- *Sing praises of Caring Science concepts: being-in-relation and intentionality*
- *Give voice to spiritual caring and my experiences of nursing in Ukraine*

## ■ JOURNEY TO CARING SCIENCE AND CARITAS

I have been a registered nurse for over 40 years. I was one of the lucky ones. I always wanted to be a nurse and have never been unhappy with my career choice. I have worked as a staff nurse, a research assistant, and a databank manager. I have been a nurse clinical specialist, a nurse researcher, a nurse administrator, and an academic educator. I have worked in large teaching medical centers and small community hospitals, university settings, and small religiously affiliated liberal arts colleges. In eight different states and four regions of the United States, I have been privileged to touch the lives of children and adults, healthy and ill, giving birth and taking their last breath. It has been a most incredible journey.

My faith has contributed in a major way to my path, and I have earnestly explored the relationship between religious beliefs, spiritual practices, and my professional nursing experiences. Being a woman of faith and of science, I strive to understand how religion and spirituality influence my physical and mental health, and how I can inspire others to include spiritual caring as a regular component of nursing practice. I have found that spiritual care is a vital element on the health/illness continuum for patients, professional and nonprofessional caregivers, and students.

My first formal introduction to nursing theory was in my master's program at the University of Pittsburgh in the early 1980s. Our professor guided us through a series of reading assignments that opened my eyes to a new world of possibilities. We eventually unleashed our creative energies in group presentations of selected theories. The one that really sticks out in my mind was a staged wedding ceremony with the bride and groom representing the marriage between theory and practice. I believe I applied theory to my personal nursing practice from that day forward.

Over the next decade I was fortunate to have attended conferences where nursing theorists were presenting their work. I was motivated by their wisdom and energized by discussions of practice application by colleagues. When I heard Dr. Jean Watson discuss her theory at a Sigma Theta Tau conference, I knew immediately that this was a match to my own beliefs and values as a nurse. She displayed the *Sacred Mirrors* of Alex Grey, a "cosmological view of the body, the mind, and the spirit" (Grey, 1990, p. 17), and I went home and ordered the book. I was inspired by the spiritual energy of the art and relished the essays by Ken Wilber. I continued to integrate conceptual approaches to practice, particularly caring leadership strategies and caring pedagogy. I reflected on the significant relationship between the art and the science of nursing and health/love/peace in the world.

These revelations contributed to my general sense of discarding the medical model for a more holistic approach to nursing care. I had several significant medical researchers as early mentors in my career and a great deal of experience with quantitative design and analysis. The transpersonal caring–healing model shifted my interest to nursing questions and I began to explore qualitative methods for the answers. The truth is that these methods were really only just beginning to be "acceptable" as scientific in the medical professions. I found that they complemented my love of literature, poetry, music, and art, which swept me into the subjective world of meaning and feeling and a multidimensional search for self. Watson's early work (1981) spoke to the quest for the whole:

> Understanding the similarities and differences between science and the humanities will help to explain why both are important in nursing and why a science of caring is needed. . . . Science is not concerned with human goals and values. Science is not necessarily concerned with individual experience and one cannot expect the sciences to keep alive a sense of common humanity. . . . The humanities are concerned with emotional responses to experiences and they look for individual difference and uniqueness. The humanities seek diversity and quality of human experiences. In the humanities, imagination and insight are validated from within the self. (p. 61)

Dr. Watson's theory touched my faith as well. It has been my experience that praying creates an envelope of peacefulness that enhances spiritual connectedness with the Divine. It is spiritual connectedness that makes the experience of prayer unique for each individual. During the act of praying, the soul or inner essence of the person is connected to a greater entity, a higher degree of consciousness, and a power that enhances transcendence and expands human possibilities. This idea is aligned closely with Watson's (1985[1979], 1988[1985], 1999, 2005, 2008) Caring Science, that the human experience of praying is intrinsically related to the coevolving human in the universe and to a sense of sacred engagement with regard to self, others, nature, and God.

I had the good fortune to study with Dr. Watson in Boulder while I was working on my dissertation. Dr. Rosemarie Rizzo Parse expertly guided my heuristic inquiry as committee chair at Loyola University Chicago (Casterline, 2006, 2009). I communicated regularly with Dr. Watson and invited her to speak at a conference in South Carolina. She asked me to become one of the original Watson Caring Science Institute (WCSI) faculty associates in 2008. I participated in the first Caritas Coach Program in Amelia Island and for the next 7 years collaborated with the caring faculty of WCSI, developing content and mentoring Caritas coaches. I became an active participant in the International Caritas Consortiums and the International Association for Human Caring. I was living Caring Science in my professional and personal life.

## ■ KEY ELEMENTS OF CARING SCIENCE AND CARITAS

My interest in spiritual health and spiritual care draw me to several specific concepts within the Caring Science framework: being-in-relation and intentionality. The transition from carative factors to the new Caritas languaging reveals a decidedly spiritual dimension and an overt message of love and caring (Watson, 2005). The success of nursing in this century will be its commitment to a covenantal ethic of human service and respect for the sacredness of life.

## BEING-IN-RELATION

Dr. Watson's (1985[1979], 1988[1985], 1999, 2005) Caring Science perspective is grounded in a relational ontology of *being-in-relation* and a worldview that acknowledges the spirit-to-spirit connection that promotes caring and loving relationships and wholeness. Relationships and connectedness allow humans to live authentically in communion with others. Furthermore, transpersonal caring relationships move beyond the ego-self and beyond the given moment to deeper connections to the spirit and with the broader universe (Watson, 1999), thus honoring the sacred within and without (Watson, 2005). Watson is explicit in supporting the concept of soul and in emphasizing the spiritual dimension of human existence. Watson's (1985[1979], 1988[1985], 1999, 2005) emphasis on the spiritual may be linked to the act of praying as a widespread spiritual practice. Both Caring Science and the act of praying emphasize the relational ontology.

A relational ontology has a foundational effect on one's ability to be self-aware, to have trusting relationships with others, and to enjoy a heart-centered communion with the sacred. My personal journey led me to self-discovery and self-care. I used mindfulness meditation and journaling to explore my inner feelings. Music was my gift and special messenger for comfort, insight, and imagination. I was called to be the choir director for my church. The sacred music and collaboration with the choir members was a mission of joy and service. Music has always contributed to my spiritual health and the richness of my relationship with God.

Teilhard de Chardin (1959) theorized the evolution of humankind moving in a specific direction of becoming, full of possibilities. Increasing complexity evolves into a progressively more conscious mind. Teilhard de Chardin posited that this evolution would eventually move man from being highly individualized, to being increasingly integrated with others/nature/the universe (1959). One imagines a giant web of conscious thought—not personal (selfish), but universal (cooperative) in its nature. Unity in love, goodwill, and peace prevails in such a universe.

In a particularly artful passage, Teilhard de Chardin speculated that people "plunge into God" by understanding that "in the *Divine Milieu* all the elements of the universe touch each other by that which is most inward and ultimate in them" (1960, p. 86). The place where "the soul is most deep and where matter is most dense" is where we are most "clearly directed, vastly expanded" and in perfect universal union. This illuminates an image that union does not mean absorbed into and lost, but that God preserves individuality. We are transfigured, but exalting in our specific attributes! Teilhard de Chardin believed that humans were created for a reason, and those defining points of our characters make up the meaningful whole. Completion in union is only available by working together with others, resulting in a communal convergence to the Omega Point.

People cannot love the Divine without loving others, and people cannot love others without moving in closer intimacy with the Divine. Spirituality is relationship. All humans are kindred spirits and love connects us with our deepest selves.

Watson views spirit as relationship and connectedness, allowing humans to live authentically and in community. Nursing care can be experienced as a sign of the spirit. Nursing *is* a spiritual relationship and an overt evocation of love and caring. Caring "tends the soul" of self and the one-being-cared-for (Watson, 1999, p. 53).

## INTENTIONALITY

*Intentionality* is defined as a mental direction or projection of awareness toward an object or outcome (Watson, 1999). Consciousness may directly or indirectly affect individual and collective well-being. Consciousness in the form of negative energy (low-frequency wavelengths) and positive energy (high-frequency wavelengths) is hypothesized to transform wholeness and influence healing possibilities. The nurse attempts to enter into and stay within the other's frame of reference, mutually searching for meaning and wholeness of being and becoming to promote comfort measures, pain control, a sense of well-being, or even spiritual transcendence of suffering. The concept of conscious intentionality paves the way toward the use of belief systems and spiritual perspectives such as imagery, visualization, prayer, and meditation practices to enhance healing and wholeness at the spiritual level of consciousness.

Prayer is a deeply personal yet profoundly universal experience. From Watson's perspective, the nurse's role in facilitating personal prayer could be seen as providing a sacred space for healing energy or the formation of a "shared consciousness, interpenetration or co-mingling of two energy fields" with the intention for healing (1999, p. 118). Prayer creates an envelope of peacefulness that enhances spiritual connectedness, making the experience of prayer unique for each individual. During the act of praying, the soul or inner essence of the person is connected to a greater entity, a higher degree of consciousness, and a power that can allow transcendence and expand human capacities. The use of reflective, subjective, and phenomenological approaches to studying prayer is congruent with Watson's interest in human experiences and meaning.

## ■ IMPLEMENTING THE THEORY IN MY WORK

My gradual self-transformation within the Caring Science paradigm, my love of the arts, and my research in spirituality and health opened an unexpected door for me in 2007. The university where I was working had been courting a relationship with a university in Ukraine. As associate dean for our school of nursing, I joined three other faculty members on a visit to Ternopil State Medical University (TSMU), where we shared education strategies, administrative policies, and laboratory equipment with the TSMU School of Nursing faculty. Their director, Dr. Nataliya Lishchenko, became a close friend and colleague. In 2008, Dr. Lishchenko taught at our university in the United States and then immigrated to Toronto, Canada, where she became a community health nurse. We traveled to Ukraine together twice after that, participating in professional nursing activities and conducting research.

Ukraine, located in Eastern Europe, is the second largest country in Europe in terms of land mass (slightly larger than Texas). Ukraine has a population of 46.4 million, with 75% ethnic Ukrainians. Kiev is the capital of Ukraine, a bustling modern city of government and commerce. Almost the entire country of Ukraine is a flat plain, with elevations generally below 350 m. The Carpathian Mountains intrude at the extreme west, with the Crimean Peninsula on the southern coast; this area was recently annexed by Russia. The recent political upheavals have caused a crisis in the already struggling Ukrainian economy. Ukrainian nationalism is strong. Ukrainian Orthodox Christianity and Russian Orthodox are primarily practiced in Ukraine today.

## NURSING IN UKRAINE

When I was there, Ukraine had over 433,000 nurses, and 70% held associate's and bachelor's degrees in nursing. Others were midwives, lab and dental technicians, and so-called "pheldshers" (equivalent of physician assistants in the United States). The ratio between physicians and nurses in Ukraine was 1:2.2.

Like many places in the world, there is a shortage of nurses and physicians in Ukraine. Many professionals are leaving Ukraine for better salaries elsewhere. There were 122 state-owned nursing schools in Ukraine, financed through state and local budgets. In 2007, 24,667 students were enrolled into nursing programs statewide (N. Lishchenko, personal communication, 2008). Master's education for nurses and professional associations was initiated in 2008 by the Chief Specialist for Human Resources, Education and Science of Ministry of Public Health of Ukraine, a champion for nursing education. There were many international collaborative projects with programs in Europe and the United States to improve nursing education and community long-term care.

The inpatient health care system was organized into three levels: rural catchment hospitals, with very basic inpatient facilities (3.5% of all hospital beds); municipal and central district hospitals (70% of all hospital beds); and regional and supra-regional specialization (25% of all hospital beds).

## EXPLORING CARING

On my second trip to Ukraine, I was invited as a keynote speaker for the International Nursing Conference on "Philosophy in Nursing" at the picturesque Chervona Kalyna retreat and conference center outside of Ternopil. There were more than 150 delegates from 120 Ukrainian Nursing Schools, clinics, and hospitals from all over the country, as well as some medical universities with nursing faculty. Of course, I spoke about Caring Science and presented a book authored by Dr. Jean Watson to the chief specialist for nursing education. It was one of the most amazing days of my life and the nurses shared many stories with me about their caring practices.

After the conference, Dr. Lishchenko and I conducted a quantitative study approved by the university Institutional Review Board (IRB) of Ukrainian nurses at two major medical centers in Ternopil, using the Coates' Caring Efficacy Scale. We received permission to use the scale and Dr. Lishchenko translated it into Ukraine. Seventy-five nurses agreed to answer the survey, ages ranging from 20 to 60 with an average age of 35. Their average years of experience was 16, ranging from 1 to 39 years. The aggregate caring scores revealed similar perceptions of caring in this sample of Ukrainian staff nurses (4.89) as previously reported by Coates for nurses in the United States (4.9).

We asked the nurses to tell us a story about a transpersonal caring moment. One nurse shared the following:

> In 10 years of my work in surgical department I have had several moments like this. The most recent I am going to remember all my life. It is about a 40-year-old woman, who was admitted to our hospital after sexual abuse and rape. She had major surgery and was expecting several more surgeries. She was a single mother, raising two children. All our staff in the department were so passionate and caring. We tried to do even more than we can for her, every heart was touched by her story. I remember a boarding school worker coming with her two children to visit her (children were temporarily placed into the boarding school until her condition stabilized). It was so painful to see that. We'll remember this woman for a long time.

Another story was shared from a neurosurgery rehabilitation nurse.

> I've seen many situations in my 5 years of nursing experience. However, the most memorable was the day, when we admitted a very young man with a spinal injury. He spent near two months in our unit, was not able to move his arms or legs and was on a ventilator most of the time he spent with us. I remember his desperate parents, who had this strong belief that their son is going to make it. They never stopped praying for him. That particular situation was very difficult, but we went through it all together. The parents of this young man still believe that their son will be walking. They go to the rehabilitation sanatorium, they

take care of him with all their efforts, they want him to be healthy. And we as the nursing staff that was involved in his treatment in our unit keep connections with them and are ready to help them in any way.

## PRAYING RESEARCH

On our last trip to Ukraine together, Dr. Lishchenko and I went on a pilgrimage to the Carpathian Mountains. It was a beautiful summer and the mountains were brimming with wildflowers and raspberries. God was everywhere. We visited a music museum full of folk instruments and a pysanky (eggs ornately decorated using a hot wax method) museum. We climbed to a hilltop cabin where we leafed through hundreds of personal journals kept by a woman who sat at her window every day and reflected her gratitude to God for her life and the beautiful mountains. Along many hiking paths we would discover small wooden prayer houses used by the locals before and after work. The prayer houses had hand-painted walls and ceilings, carved woodwork, and were filled with icons of saints, religious art, bibles, and poetry. They were reminders of the importance of faith in these communities.

When we returned refreshed from the mountains, we proceeded with our study about the experience of prayer (Casterline & Lishchenko, 2009). We recruited six women who agreed to tell us about their experiences with praying. Three of them spoke English and three of them told their story in Ukrainian, which Nataliya translated for me. Using the heuristic inquiry method, I explicated depictions for each participant. I offer the following examples:

> The act of praying for Svetlana was influenced by a promise to pray daily in return for her son's health. She feels a natural and joyful connection with a larger presence and is grateful that she is not alone in the universe. Praying improves her health, particularly when she communicates with the saints.

> The act of praying for Olga occurs when sharing her deepest feelings through informal dialogue with God. She is relieved in the knowledge that God is always listening. When she feels the closeness of the Holy Spirit, the atmosphere becomes calm and she experiences a lightness of her soul.

A composite depiction blends the participant's stories into a whole.

> The act of praying is a daily sharing of sincere thoughts and needs with a God who is always listening. A close connection is enhanced through the power of saints and icons. Divine guidance and protection offers feelings of calm, relief, health, lightness of soul, courage, and joy.

Findings in heuristic inquiry are ultimately represented by a creative synthesis, an original interaction of the data reflecting the researcher's intuition, imagination,

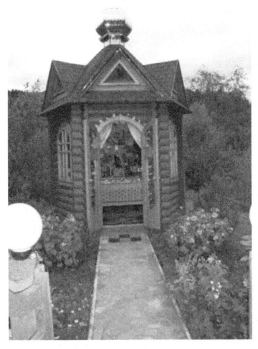

FIGURE 11.1   Country prayer house in the Carpathian Mountains.

and personal knowledge of the meaning of the experience. This might be a poem or sculpture or music—any art form. In this study, the creative synthesis took the form of a country prayer house in the Carpathian Mountains (Figure 11.1).

## ■ CONCLUSION

As Robert Frost envisioned is his 1943 poem, "Choose Something Like a Star," individuals are passionately aware that the search for wisdom and eternal truth extends far beyond themselves (Poirier & Richardson, 1995). A widespread commitment to holistic care and the timeless ethic of caring–healing relationships is required. Health of the human spirit includes caring for the unobservable, intangible element of human spirituality. Watson's postmodern, transpersonal view considers person as spirit, soul energy as sacred energy, and the body as the instrument of the soul (1999). This new, emerging cosmology calls for a sense of reverence and sacredness with regard to life and all living things, acknowledging a convergence between art, science, and spirituality.

## ■ ACKNOWLEDGMENT

The author kindly acknowledges the assistance of Dr. Nataliya Lishchenko.

# ■ REFERENCES

Casterline, G. L. (2006). The experience of the act of praying. (Doctoral dissertation, Loyola University Chicago, 2006). *Dissertation Abstracts International, 67,* 1915.

Casterline, G. L. (2009). Heuristic inquiry: Artistic science for nursing. *Southern Online Journal for Nursing Research, 9*(1), 1–8.

Casterline, G. L., & Lishchenko, N. (2009). Nursing in Ukraine: A survey of caring behaviors. *Nursing: Ukrainian Scientific and Practical Journal, 2,* 9–13.

Grey, A. (1990). *Sacred mirrors: The visionary art of Alex Grey.* Rochester, VT: Inner Traditions International.

Poirier, R., & Richardson, M. (Eds). (1995). *Frost: Collected poems, prose, & plays.* New York, NY: Library of America.

Teilhard de Chardin, P. (1959). *The phenomenon of man.* London, England: William Collins Sons.

Teilhard de Chardin, P. (1960). *The divine milieu.* London, England: William Collins Sons.

Watson, J. (1981). Some issues related to a science of caring for nursing practice. In M. M. Leininger (Ed.), *Caring: An essential human need* (pp. 61–67). Detroit, MI: Wayne State Press.

Watson, J. (1985[1979]). *Nursing: The philosophy and science of caring.* Boulder, CO: University Press of Colorado. (Original work published 1979, Brown and Company.)

Watson, J. (1988[1985]). *Nursing: Human science and human care. A theory of nursing.* Norwalk, CT: Appleton-Century-Crofts [Reprinted 1988, New York, NY: National League for Nursing]. (Original work published 1985, Appleton-Century-Crofts.)

Watson, J. (1999). *Postmodern nursing and beyond.* London, England: Churchill Livingstone.

Watson, J. (2005). *Caring science as sacred science.* Philadelphia, PA: F.A. Davis.

Watson, J. (2008). *Nursing: The philosophy and science of caring.* Boulder, CO: University of Colorado Press.

# CHAPTER TWELVE

# Seeing the Person Through the Patient: A Human Caring Reference Model for Health Care and Research

*Sandra Vacchi*

---

**CARITAS QUOTE**

*A person may have an illness or even disease that is completely hidden from our eyes. To find solutions it is necessary to find meanings. A person's human predicament may not be related to the external world as much as to the person's inner world as he or she experiences it. (Watson, 2012, p. 63)*

---

*After learning about the Theory of Human Caring by Dr. Jean Watson, a group of nurses in Italy is advancing Human Caring Science through practice, education, and research. They have formed a research group, established a website, sponsored conferences, and are challenging the medical establishment with a first-of-its-kind initiative in Caring Science in Italy. This chapter tells their story and their journey to study nurses', nursing students', and patients' experiences with caring.*

■ OBJECTIVES

*The objectives of this chapter are to:*

• *Describe the process used to conduct nursing research aimed at measuring the level of human caring within different health care systems*

- *Identify the most appropriate instrument for the Italian culture to evaluate the present level of caring*
- *Contribute to a scientifically approved methodology*

## ■ JOURNEY TO CARING SCIENCE AND CARITAS LITERACY

Italian nurses are becoming increasingly aware of the need for theories that describe global phenomena as well as instruments that enable direct evaluation. As a consequence, conceptual models and theories are becoming important frames of reference for nurses, nursing students, and other health sciences colleagues in Italy. This chapter describes the adoption and spread of Caring Science in Italy, including the methods and findings of a qualitative and quantitative study in which the author and her colleagues were mentored by Dr. Jean Watson.

## ■ A JOURNEY BEGUN 10 YEARS AGO

For many years, nursing knowledge has been influenced by a medical–clinical approach to curing. This approach led to the separation of the mind–body–spirit; the body prevails as the focus. This Cartesian model of science eliminates any sense of spirit and detaches the humans from their environment and from each other, reducing the human being to an object. A *one-way clinical vision* leaves nursing to set aside its original professional purpose of taking care of humans and humanity in a global and holistic sense.

The nursing curricula in Italy include nursing theories, one of which is the Theory of Human Caring by Dr. Watson. While other theories are principally based on *doing,* Dr. Watson's theory presents an existential phenomenological perspective. Watson believes holistic nursing requires a deep knowledge about nursing art. Through the study of humanistic topics, our minds are opened and our reflective abilities enhanced to contribute to our personal growth.

Traditionally, hospital nursing was more inclined toward *doing* and focused on clinical needs. Health care is hospital centered and medically oriented. It was not customary or easy to speak about patients' authentic needs. Nurses also had a dependent role in the past, asking physicians for permission before doing something for their patients. Fortunately, nursing practice and health care in Italy are evolving, taking on a more holistic vision. How could we really understand the meaning of *being a nurse*? How could we learn the confidence to stand alone, the courage to make tough decisions, and the compassion to listen to others' needs? Growth requires nourishment through new knowledge that provides a holistic way of seeing, understanding, and approaching others' practice.

If we change, everything around us changes. Nursing is a personal commitment and nursing practice is the visible expression of our professional knowledge. Also, nursing is a manifestation of our intention, consciousness, approach, and feelings when we care for another person: "We learn to recognize ourselves in others by engaging in a transpersonal caring moment" (Watson, 1985, p. 59). So, we can discover an inner path of transformation in practice when guided by caring and healing.

Over the years, Dr. Watson has visited Italy and Europe many times to facilitate the continued professional growth of nurses and other professionals in Caring Science:

- The First National Congress: *La Disciplina Infermieristica: il vivere quotidiano nella continuità assistenziale fra Ospedale, Famiglia e Comunità,* Almese-Torino, Italy, 2007
- Intensive Seminar and Coaching (reserved for our research group): *Theory—Research of Human Caring and Assessment of Caring,* Torino, Italy, 2009
- *Italian Nurses United in Human Caring,* Lucca, 2013
- *Uniting European Nurses and Health Science Colleagues in Human Caring,* Torino, Italy, 2014
- *European Caritas Seminar and Retreat,* Lucca, Italy, 2015
- Conference: *La relation humaniste, un garant de la qualité et la securité des soins,* Polé de Recherche Innovation en soins et professionalisation—Institut et Haute Ecole de La Santé La Source, Lausanne, Switzerland, 2015

Moreover, the Caring in Progress International Association worked to extend research, practice, and teaching of Caring Science to nurses and other professionals, helping to develop new knowledge of human caring to transform nursing, education, and practice.

I met Dr. Watson 10 years ago. Since then, I have worked to learn more about her theory and philosophy. I have had several opportunities to spend time with Dr. Watson at presentations and meetings. Most recently, in October 2015, I attended the International Caritas Consortium in Onalaska, Wisconsin, where I presented our research findings (Vacchi, Guiotto, Gurlino, Poponi, & Vinassa, 2009). I am currently participating in the Caritas Coach Education Program (CCEP), sponsored by the Watson Caring Science Center, University of Colorado. Each face-to-face meeting with Dr. Watson furthers my knowledge and brings a stronger connection to caring and Caritas healing. Thus, through caring we can really make a difference.

## ■ A SMALL GROUP INSPIRED BY A FIRM CONVICTION

In 2009, a small group of colleagues and I decided to work directly with Dr. Watson and the Watson Caring Science Institute (WCSI). We formed a research group with the intention of conducting research studies in human caring theory as experienced in professional nursing practice. A project was initiated based on the firm belief that the purpose of health professions, above all nursing, is *to take care of* another person, not only *to be near another person*. Professionals who *take care of* cannot ignore the consciousness of the transpersonal relationship that is essential in the caring–healing process.

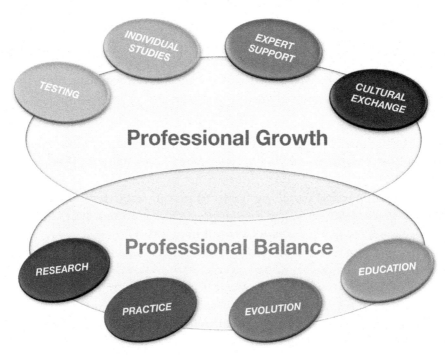

FIGURE 12.1 Professional growth and balance.
*Source:* Vacchi (2015).

*Doing* and *being* are not separate actions belonging to different horizons but moments of the same behavior; this is why nurses perceive these elements of *reading the body as a biography-subject* and not as pathology. We have also been inspired by the firm conviction that *caring* is already practiced even if we are not fully aware of it; however, if duly measured, it can be perceived within the framework of Human Caring Science. Thus, we aimed to identify a framework that would help us recognize both caring and uncaring behaviors in nursing practice and, subsequently, to use our findings to improve practice with an eye toward healing–caring.

Our qualitative/quantitative research represents a unique and historical milestone as the first nursing research in Italy supported and directed by Dr. Watson. The utmost importance of this mentorship indeed represented the deep support for our entire research project. The work adhered to the research guidelines provided by Dr. Watson, serving as the vademecum of the group during the research process.

## ■ OUR APPROACH

We approached our research from two points of view—professional development and professional balance (Figure 12.1). By way of professional development, we taught ourselves as much as possible about caring and the Theory of Human Caring through:

**Testing.** We needed to check ourselves and our knowledge, skills, and ability in using [and] managing some topics about the model and research instruments.

**Individual Studies.** We focused on the analysis of the original texts in their native language: *Nursing: Human Science and Human Care: A Theory of Nursing* (Watson, 1985); *Nursing: Philosophy and Science of Caring* (Watson, 2008b); *Postmodern Nursing and Beyond* (Watson, 1999); *Assessing and Measuring Caring in Nursing and Health Science* (Watson, 2002, 2008a); reading original text selected on a specific subject; using the official website of the WCSI.

**Expert Support.** We contacted Dr. Jean Watson through the WCSI and developed our research methodology with her, which became for us and our work an authoritative and prestigious opportunity.

**Cultural Exchange.** We used reference patterns that allowed for a global background description of the phenomena and specific instruments that enabled direct practical application.

Our second point of view was professional balance through which we continued learning through these steps:

**Education.** In our coaching project with the support of Dr. Jean Watson, we obtained detailed knowledge about the project's theme. We learned more about the research measurement tools in order to be able to select the best one to survey the Italian culture. Finally, we learned how to implement the model into professional practice.

**Evolution.** We began by internalizing that

> . . . if a profession doesn't have its own language, it doesn't exist; thus it's important to name, claim, articulate and act upon the phenomena of nursing and caring if nursing is to fulfill its mandate for society. This includes taking mature professional responsibility for giving voice to, standing up for and acting on its knowledge, values, ethics and skilled practice of caring, healing and health. (Watson, 2008b, p. 4)

**Practice.** We merged and summarized Caring Science as [a] basic model to create a new culture that is *heart centered* and *gives a body* becoming for self, other, and systems in our health structures.

**Research.** We made decisions about the research sites and methodology (who, what, when, where, how, and why). We revised our methods and reconsidered our research sites (institutional revision and access) by answering the questions of who, what, when, where, how, and why.

## ■ A METHODOLOGY TO START UP

At this point, we assessed the project's feasibility and evaluated where we could conduct our research in health care and educational systems (institutional revision and access). We decided to evaluate the level of caring as perceived by patients, nurses, and nursing students (who). The goal was to estimate the perception of caring, referring to the theoretical and conceptual model of Dr. Watson (what). We kept systematic records of the chronology of the project (when). We selected three sites in which to conduct our research: hospital, home, and university (where). We decided to include patients, nurse, and nursing students.

Throughout the research planning, using measurement tools referred to the model and analyzing sample size, data, and results, we chose the most important outcomes for nursing practice and started the discussion about the results (how). Our goal was to increase the caring level by nurses and health science colleagues, as well as students (why).

The convenience sample consisted of 165 subjects: 27 hospital and home care patients, 28 hospital and home care nurses, and 110 students from Università dell'Insubria, Varese, Regione Lombardia.

## ■ CLARIFYING THE WAY TO CARING: FROM BIOCIDIC TO BIOGENIC ENVIRONMENTS

We selected the Caring Patient Assessment Scale (CPAS) on the advice of Dr. Watson. Using a forward and reverse-translation process, the instrument was translated into Italian for the first time reflecting five of the Caritas Processes—essential points of the theory: (1) loving-kindness, (4) helping–trusting relationship, (8) healing environment, (9) holistic care, (10) spiritual/mysterious and unknown existential dimensions. These five items explained 78% of the variance. The Italian version of CPAS was approved by Dr. Watson and included the logo of the WCSI (Figure 12.2).

The Italian CPAS contained a five-item Likert-type scale ranging from never, rarely, occasionally, frequently, to always. Scores were interpreted according to Halldorsdottir's model (1991) where caring was categorized at the higher end of the responses as life giving = biogenic and life sustaining = bioactive. The mid-range was classified as life neutral = biopassive. Uncaring was categorized at the lower end of the responses: life restraining = biostatic, life destroying = biocidic (Hallsdorsdottir's model as found in Watson, 2008b; Figure 12.3).

Patient subjects were selected based on age (adults), length of stay (at least 1 week), and ability to read and write. The CPAS was administered in paper form the day before discharge by a person not involved in the care of the patient. The project was approved by the ethics committee for human subject research (Figure 12.4).

The final CPAS results from patients included:

- Biocidic = 0%
- Biostatic = 2%
- Biopassive = 7%
- Bioactive = 21%
- Biogenic = 70% of patients reported experiencing a biogenic interaction with their nurses

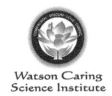

Watson Caring
Science Institute

## Caring Patient Assessment Score
### (Rilevamento del Caring – Paziente)

**Istruzioni:** Nel rispondere alle domande, per favore consideri l'assistenza complessiva ricevuta durante il ricovero ospedaliero.

Crocettare, per ciascuna descrizione, **la risposta più onesta**

| Durante la mia permanenza in Ospedale: | Mai | Raramente | Occasionalmente | Frequentemente | Sempre |
|---|---|---|---|---|---|
| Gli infermieri provvedono costantemente alla mia assistenza con gentilezza amorevole | | | | | |
| Gli infermieri si relazionano con me in quanto persona completa, aiutandomi a prendermi cura delle mie necessità e a gestire le mie preoccupazioni | | | | | |
| Gli infermieri instaurano, nei miei confronti, una relazione d'aiuto e di fiducia | | | | | |
| Gli infermieri creano un ambiente favorevole alla guarigione nel rispetto dell'interezza del mio corpo, della mente e dello spirito | | | | | |
| Gli infermieri accettano e rispettano le mie credenze, che possono concorrere alla guarigione per me e la mia famiglia | | | | | |

- Consiglierebbe il nostro Ospedale a qualcuno che Le sta a cuore?

          ❏  SI          ❏  NO

- Nell'apprezzare la Sua disponibilità, La invitiamo a voler condividere, qui di seguito, i momenti importanti d'assistenza o "mancata assistenza" che ha vissuto durante la Sua permanenza in Ospedale

_____
_____
_____
_____

**Un sincero GRAZIE per la condivisione e per aver contribuito al nostro lavoro di ricerca**

FIGURE 12.2   Caring Patient Assessment Score. Copyright 2009 by Watson Caring Science Institute.

Adapted from Nelson, Watson, and InovaHealth (2009).

Translated by: Sandra Vacchi, Annachiara Guiotto, Cinzia Poponi, and Stefania Gurlino (Torino, Italy).

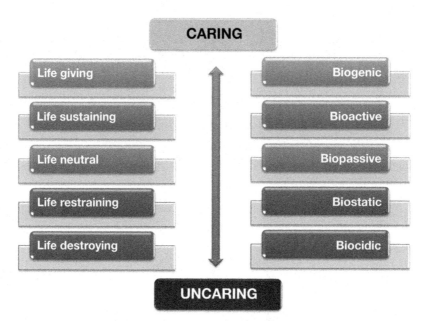

FIGURE 12.3   Caring–uncaring relationship.
Adapted from Vacchi (2015).
*Source:* Halldorsdottir (1991).

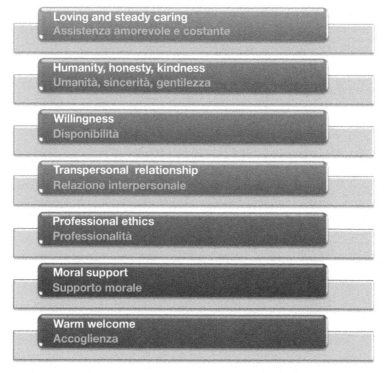

FIGURE 12.4   Connection between open narrative data and key words.
*Source:* Vacchi (2015).

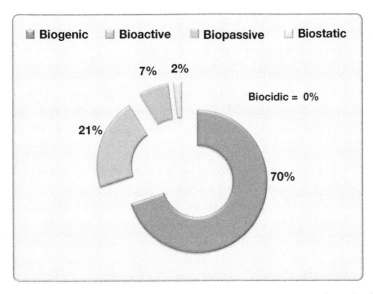

FIGURE 12.5   Patients/nurses relationship—survey percentage related to biocidic/biogenic model.

*Source:* Vacchi (2015).

TABLE 12.1   **Caring/Caritas Relationship Categories**

| Patients' Key Words of Open Data | Referred to Caritas Process Number |
|---|---|
| Loving and steady caring | 1 |
| Humanity, honesty, compassion | 8 |
| Willingness | 7 |
| Transpersonal relationship | 4 |
| Professional ethics | 6 |
| Moral support | 5 |
| Warm welcome | 2 |

*Source:* Vacchi (2015).

The results confirmed our hypothesis—caring is already practiced by nurses even if it does not exactly align with Dr. Watson's Theory of Human Caring. Furthermore, patients' experience of caring corresponds to mainly (91%) a bioactive or biogenic level (Figure 12.5).

The findings support the Caritas Processes (Table 12.1).

We also examined nurses' and nursing students' qualitative responses. In their view:

• The patient is frequently considered as a body and not as a human being.
• There is a lack of global human caring between members of the health care team toward the patient.

- There is not enough time to be completely present and express a caring relationship.
- There is discomfort associated with end of life.

Patients often recognize nurses' skilled approach but nurses are doubtful about their ability of being and becoming, of moving toward a *bioactive/biogenic* condition. It is, I believe, possible to start a path of engagement, the four paths toward caring and healing, as adapted by Dr. Watson from Fox (1991) and Arrien (1993):

- *Via Negativa*—From "daring the dark," we can put new light on our obstacles and difficulties. (Watson, 2005, p. 232)
- *Via Positiva*—Once we open to the via positive, we can find caring moments of joy and beauty, grace and gratitude, throughout all our day, every day . . . offer human contact, human-to-human connection, creating healing environments, . . . creating spaces and professional culture whereby caring-healing practices flourish. . . . (Watson, 2005, p. 233)
- *Via Creativa*—On this path we plumb new, deeper dimensions of self and our unique gifts and talents that we can offer as compassionate service on behalf of others. (Watson, 2005, p. 234)
- *Via Transformativa*—From this via . . . we hold sacred space for caring-healing at all levels while letting go of outcomes, open to outcomes that may never be predicted nor controlled from conventional views of leadership. . . . (Watson, 2005, p. 235)

We need to grow and nurture our profession and ourselves and drive our efforts toward small words of kindness, consciousness, and more self-confidence, our way of being silent, of looking, of speaking, and of acting. And we are already on this journey.

## ■ CONCLUSION

Reflecting on the message that Dr. Watson offered to us in Turin, Italy, in 2009—"This one moment for this one person . . ."— we connect it with the fact that work, every single work, is empty without love. Thus, we need to put passion in our work, little drops of passion that find a gentle slope to come out; this passion can take root and grow up in our lives. Like drops of water, it becomes clear and more evident in the way we nurture it, putting breath in our spirits in everything we do; that means to put a little piece of our own being in what we accomplish at work and in our lives every day.

## ■ REFERENCES

Arrien, A. (1993). *The four-fold way: Walking the paths of the warrior, teacher, healer, and visionary.* San Francisco, CA: Harper.

Fox, M. (1991). *Creation spirituality: Liberating gifts for the peoples of the Earth.* San Francisco, CA: Harper.

Hallorsdottir, S. (1991). Five basic modes of being with another. In D. Gaut & M. Leininger (Eds.), *Caring: The compassionate healer* (pp. 37–50). New York, NY: National League for Nursing.

Nelson, J., Watson J., & InovaHealth. (2009). Caring Factor Survey (CFS). In J. Watson (Ed.), *Assessing and measuring caring in nursing and health science* (2nd ed., pp. 253–258). New York, NY: Springer Publishing.

Vacchi, S. (2015, October). *An Italian research aimed at implementing the caring in nursing practice: Adopting and adapting the Caritas Patient Score Survey.* Paper presented at the meeting of the 21st International Caritas Consortium, Onalaska, WI.

Vacchi, S., Guiotto, A., Gurlino, S., Poponi, C., & Vinassa, B. (2009). *Patients' survey hospital/day care governance experience aimed at implementing the human caring model in the professional nursing practice.* District Health Care Research Project Scientific Report, Turin, Italy.

Watson, J. (1985). *Nursing: Human science and human care: A theory of nursing.* Norwalk: CT: Appleton-Century-Crofts.

Watson, J. (1999). *Postmodern nursing and beyond.* Edinburgh, Scotland: Churchill-Livingstone.

Watson, J. (2002). *Assessing and measuring caring in nursing and health science.* New York, NY: Springer Publishing.

Watson, J. (2005). *Caring science as sacred science.* Philadelphia, PA: F.A. Davis.

Watson, J. (2008a). *Assessing and measuring caring in nursing and health science* (2nd ed.). New York, NY: Springer Publishing.

Watson, J. (2008b). *Nursing: Philosophy and science of caring* (Rev. ed.). Boulder, CO: University Press of Colorado.

Watson, J. (2012). *Human caring science. A theory of nursing* (2nd ed.). Sudbury, MA: Jones & Bartlett.

# PART FIVE

# *Caritas Praxis*

This section begins with two South African authors who are linking the concept of caring with the traditional South African concept of *Ubuntu*. Dr. Charlenè Downing, currently a postdoctoral fellow in the Watson Caring Science Institute, conducted an integrative review on the subject of Albertina Nontsikelelo Sisulu, activist and nurse in South Africa who embodied caring. Dr. Downing plans to use appreciative inquiry to explore and describe the best caring moments of fourth-year student nurses. Our second author, also from the University of Johannesburg and a postdoctoral fellow in the Watson Caring Science Institute, Dr. Anna Nolte, Caritas Coach, describes her plan to develop a conceptual model of midwifery for South Africa based on Caring Science, scholarship that will also be linked to Ubuntu. Dr. Joseph Giovannoni, a Caring Science Scholar and postdoctoral fellow in the Watson Caring Science Institute, describes an emerging practice of caring within a group he calls "Society's Safe-Keepers," interprofessionals—rehabilitation and parole officers—who can be positive caring role models and uphold human dignity to those who have violated the rights and human dignity of others. In his novel work, Dr. Giovannoni advocates a caring and compassionate approach to perpetrators while holding them accountable. Maryanne Sandberg, a nursing educator from Georgia, United States, provides an inspiring clinical narrative where she, as nurse, was the energetic field for caring–healing, using all ways of knowing/ being/doing/becoming for a young man with a rare genetic disorder so that he could live a life of meaning and joy.

# CHAPTER THIRTEEN

# Practices of Caring: A South African Perspective

*Charlenè Downing*

*The chapter highlights my current relationship with caring through the South African lens of Ubuntu. I guide you on my journey of being part of and living in the world of caring. The chapter begins with the world of my caring and how I live and believe to work with and be in the conscious space of caring toward myself and all others who enter and are part of my journey. I am a postdoctoral fellow in Caring Science with Dr. Jean Watson.*

## ■ OBJECTIVES

*The objectives of this chapter are to:*

- *Illuminate my living as an evolving human being in the Caring Science world*
- *Illustrate ways of application in the South African context*
- *Demonstrate the application of Caring Science within appreciative inquiry*

## ◼ JOURNEY TO CARING SCIENCE AND CARITAS LITERACY

See beauty in all, and see caring happening . . . a mindful approach towards the seeing, believing, thinking, and feeling of beauty in all we do.

Wearing the caring motto "in your heart" enables me to make conscious decisions to be a concerned and participative listener when someone talks to me, giving the person the platform to promote the communication and listen and reflect with attention. For me it is more in how I am with . . . the genuineness of my attention to the individual and they feel my presence in the caring moment. To care is part of my living space.

Caring is close to my heart. I have so many persons in my world who teach me about caring and show me the value of deep caring and the fulfilling shift in my heart to know that I cared at multiple levels and moments during the course of the day. Acts of kindness toward all people is a principle that is applied throughout my day and there are days that I horribly fail or miss the moment. At the end of the day, I take stock and then reintegrate and ignite my ability and heart, yearning to care the next day.

I ask the following questions during my stock taking:

- How did I do?
- How can I do?
- Where did the engagement with the caring moment come from? My heart or my head?
- What do I take with me for the next day? Blessings for the beauty of the caring moment and individuals that engaged with me to develop and sustain the loving, open, and caring moments of engagement.
- Did I use the caring moments given to me? And did I take the caring moments to the fullest of care?
- How did I care for myself today? This is crucial for me, as I can only contribute and evolve in caring when I feel and know that I am cared for. Reflection of self in a quiet time period every morning and evening also brought about the being of caring. . . . Sometimes just to be with the person in the moment.

I have a deep and committed caring to humanity and the optimization for the persons involved in the caring process. I share a deep awareness of the changes in caring, more environmental . . . the trend of aggression, uncaring attitudes between professional nurses and students, and students' changes in their perceptions of role models. I grew up with role models, and to this day I can remember their names, see their faces, and have a deep emotional tie with how they contributed to my world of getting to know about caring.

Caring is the critical essence of nursing, the main ingredient. If one should move and use the metaphor of baking a cake, you will have no cake without caring or it might be true that you will have a very bland, mediocre cake. This gap that I felt made me aware of my relationship with students, being in a critical position to develop and sustain loving, trusting–caring relationships (Caritas Process #4; Watson, 2008).

## ■ KEY ELEMENTS OF CARING SCIENCE AND CARITAS

Caring happens in the moment where one sees or feels the moment to act from the heart with *loving-kindness, compassion,* and *equanimity with self and others* (Caritas Process #1; Watson, 2008). In the moment of caring, I engage in being authentically present, enabling the person to *see hope, be hope,* and *hold the belief that hope is attainable* (Caritas Process #2; Watson, 2008).

I am in a position to enhance the lives of students at an undergraduate, post-basic, and postgraduate level; critical to my heart is to see and seek the beauty in each of the students. I am seeing the beauty of each caring moment beyond the broken, worn, and bent aspects within the connection, seeking, feeling, hearing, and being part of and present within the beauty and/or brokenness. Therefore, being in the moment with a consciousness to embrace and appreciate the sharing of laughter, tears, deep regret, and/or guilt, all of the emotions and many more . . . to be with the brokenness and find a lens or get to a clear vision to see the beauty and/or brokenness and beyond.

History plays a central role in my life. I love detailed, in-depth description and understanding the influence of life and living. One remarkable woman is an integral part of my living and being as a South African. Her name is Albertina Nontsikelelo Sisulu—she is celebrated in the spirit of great nurses. In the world of caring and nursing, it would be nursing and nurses who provide the connectedness to the persons in need of care and hope. It is nursing and nurses who instill hope and trust, and nursing provides the most excellent and competent care possible in those critical moments of engagement with our patients. Albertina Sisulu, also known as "the mother of the nation," activist and nurse, led a selfless and courageous life: unwavering commitment to a nonracial philosophy of human equality and dignity for all in common society throughout her long and eventful life. I highlight just a few aspects of this most legendary woman as a nurse. The following points are taken from the South African History Online website (South African History Online, n.d.).

- After growing up in Transkei, she started her general training in 1940 at the old Jo'burg Gen (Johannesburg General), now known as Hillbrow Hospital.
- Albertina was shocked at the poor intercollegial relationships between nurses, which were displayed on a racial basis. Six months into Albertina's training she witnessed an incident that led to inequality of care and dignity on the basis of the ethnicity of the patients.
- Her mother's death in 1941 escalated further memories of uncaring. The hospital matron would not allow Albertina to return home to mourn her mother's death.

- In 1944, Albertina married her fiance, Walter. Nelson Mandela, also called Madiba, was their best man and Albertina's friend Evelyn (Madiba's first wife and also a nurse) was one of the bridesmaids. She qualified as a nurse in the same year.
- In 1954, Albertina obtained her midwifery qualification and she was employed by the City Health of Johannesburg. The job raised challenges; for example, Albertina had to travel on foot to visit her patients in townships. She used to carry her suitcase full of her apparatus (bottles, lotions, bowls, and receivers) on her head.
- During 1958, the South African Nursing Council demanded that all nurses and student nurses supply their identity numbers to the Council. Following a demonstration by a delegation of nurses, the Council dropped the demand for identity numbers.
- She educated and supported a family and an extended family on a nurse's salary for most of her life.
- Elinor Sisulu said:
  > I never failed to be amazed by the way Albertina coped with a workload that would exhaust most people half her age. After a full day at the surgery, she would return home to find local activists waiting to see her. Most days of the week, she would face another three to four hours of meetings before going to bed. Her weekends were also mostly taken up with meetings and frequent interviews with local and overseas journalists, many of whom were interested in the mobilisation of women under apartheid. (Sisulu, 2003; South African History Online, n.d.)
- The University of Johannesburg conferred an honorary doctorate degree on Albertina in acknowledgment of her revolutionary role in the pre-1994 South Africa.
- She was affectionately known as MaSisulu throughout her lifetime by the public (Downing & Hastings-Tolsma, 2016; Sisulu, 2003; South African History Online, n.d.).

Professor Marie Hastings-Tolsma and I conducted an integrative review and the full article is currently in press (Downing & Hastings-Tolsma, 2016). We completed a critical review of the available literature of caring as portrayed by Albertina Sisulu during her life within the South African context, and then further interpretation of Sisulu's work within the Ubuntu philosophy as a framework for living (Downing & Hastings-Tolsma, 2016).

Whittemore and Knafl's (2005) framework was used as the foundation for the article. We used key electronic databases, selected references, and web-based search engines for articles meeting the inclusion criteria. Eighteen nonresearch reports related to Sisulu; eight reports—three research and five nonresearch—related to Ubuntu and nursing were used for the completion of the integrative review. Data were extracted that related to relevant and conclusive best practice.

The findings of the review have the potential to provide a context for enhanced practice guidelines concerning knowledge and critical thinking about caring by nurses. Two primary factors emerged that demonstrated a culture of caring as seen through the prism of Sisuslu's life: *devoted dancer* and *creation of a healing environment*. This is a robust yet very true reflection of the African Ubuntu principles, where the focus is on the relationships between people and how these relationships should be conducted.

*The way forward would be to provide an integration of a framework for a model case development: The Albertina Sisulu way.*

The authors are in the process of developing a tentative framework for possible consideration for implementation to be tested in practice, research, and consideration as development of a practice theory. Further development of the Ubuntu and Sisulu's approach to caring would be the integration of the principles in meaningful curricula, practice patterns, and policies that emphasize caring constructs.

A short summary of integration of the Sisulu's caring and Ubuntu principles is provided. Ubuntu focuses on the "right way of living," and sharing the basic premises of Ubuntu is humanness, connectedness, cohesion, and conscience. Sisulu embraced all of these mentioned items during her life and further embroidered her life with respect, empathy, cooperation, harmony, sharing, and warmth (Downing & Hastings-Tolsma, 2016).

The life of Sisulu is portrayed by doing good as the essence of being. Caring for all and being the key thread in nursing as an art and science provides fertile ground for Human Caring Science to emerge (Hills & Watson, 2011).

The focus for the nurse is on health, healing, and caring in the patient's experience (Watson, 2008). Sisulu thus stands at the center of the caring moment and copartners nurses and patients for healing. Her focus provides a foundation for nurses to create an epicenter of caring for professional practice with patients, sharing human experiences, happenings, and encounters in a conscious interaction of *now*. Incorporating Sisulu's principles within the context of Ubuntu moves the "good" to the wider practice field of caring. The philosophy of human freedom, living the choice of caring in a mindfulness in everyday living, is thus important (Downing & Hastings-Tolsma, 2016).

In the spirit of Ubuntu and the life of Sisulu, the practice of loving-kindness, creating an enabling environment of faith and sensitivity to self and other to develop authentic relationships, is critical.

I revisit the relationship about living and being caring and move to how we teach and transfer caring. A project that is part of the caring focus and part of my journey as a postdoctoral student with Dr. Jean Watson is *Best Practices of Caring* through the eyes of student nurses. The focus of the study is embedded in the following research questions:

- How can appreciative inquiry (AI) with student nurses assist in exploring and describing best caring moments?
- What can be done to further create a culture of caring in student nurses?

The nursing profession continues to struggle with the complexity and dynamics involved in providing competent, caring professionals to render patient care of a high standard and to work in a healthy practice environment.

Caring forms an integral part of nursing and is demonstrated throughout the practice and learning of nursing. Caring is the assistance given to another person to help him or her grow to be more within himself or herself. Nursing is a caring practice whereby the nurse engages with the patient during caring moments across the illness–health and well-being continuum (Moody & Pesut, 2006). Nursing is thus a relationship-centered partnership and embraces caring as an interpersonal relationship. A caring educational environment is related to the learning, sharing, and teaching of related knowledge, skills, science, and the art of nursing. The ability of the nurse educator to convey trust, confidence, and caring through individualized attention to student nurses is essential in a teaching and learning partnership. Nurse educators are committed to teaching student nurses about nursing and caring through this teaching and learning relationship. Caring could therefore be viewed as a dynamic interactive process between the lecturer and student, resulting in a healthy environment of teaching and learning (Wade & Kasper, 2006).

The purpose of the study is to utilize AI to explore and describe the best caring moments of fourth-year student nurses at a higher education institution in Johannesburg. This will enable the researcher to formulate evidence-based practice guidelines to enhance the foundation of practice, study, and teaching of caring by the Department of Nursing for students during their 4 years of training to promote a culture of caring.

The research design is of a qualitative, exploratory, descriptive, and contextual design using an AI method. Phase one will consist of exploring and describing the best caring moments according to the AI method (McKeown, Fortune, & Dupuis, 2015) during which the following questions will be asked:

- What are the best caring moments while being a student in nursing? (Discovery phase)
- Thinking creatively about the future, how do you wish caring to be practiced during the training of a student nurse? (Dream phase)
- What needs to be understood in nursing education to create a culture of caring in the nursing education environment? (Design phase)
- What do we need to have in place to achieve a culture of caring in the nursing education environment? (Delivery phase)

Phase two will entail finding supporting literature applicable to the findings of the study. The strengths of the research method are to focus on affirmation, appreciation, and positive dialogue regarding the caring experiences of the student nurses. Data will be collected via social media using storyboards and discussion documents. Purposive sampling will be used in the study and data will be collected until data saturation has been reached. The data will be analyzed using thematic analysis. The principles of trustworthiness will be adhered to by ensuring credibility, confirmability, dependability, and transferability. Moreover, the researcher will abide by the ethical considerations of autonomy, beneficence, nonmaleficence, and justice.

The previously mentioned study received approval and clearance from the Higher Degree Committee of the Faculty of Health Sciences [HDC-01-01-2016] and from the Research Ethics Committee of the Faculty of Health Sciences [REC-01-04-2016], University of Johannesburg. The project is scheduled to commence within the next 4 weeks.

The findings of the study will be the first steps in creatively seeking [soul] solutions through caring practices (Caritas Process #6) and creating a healing environment at all levels (Caritas Process #8).

The attention of listening, accepting, and scientific problem solving allows for the creation of the persons who meet to be more when they leave than when they entered the engagement. Through a knowing "transfer" of giving and receiving, the caring moment of giving a piece of yourself to creatively becoming more is created.

## ■ REFERENCES

Downing, C., & Hastings-Tolsma, M. (2016). An integrative review of Albertina Sisulu and Ubuntu: Relevance to caring and nursing. *Health SA Gesondheid*. doi:10.1016/j.hsag.2016.04.002

Hills, M., & Watson, J. (2011). *Creating a caring science curriculum: An emancipatory pedagogy for nursing*. New York, NY: Springer Publishing.

McKeown, J. K. L., Fortune, D., & Dupuis, S. L. (2016). "It is like stepping into another world": Exploring the possibilities of using appreciative participatory action research to guide culture change work in community and long-term care. *Action Research, 14*, 318–334. doi:10.1177/1476750315618763

Moody, R. C., & Pesut, D. J. (2006). The motivation to care: Application and extension of motivation theory to professional nursing work. *Journal of Health Organization and Management, 20*(1), 15–48.

Sisulu, E. (2003). *Walter and Albertina Sisulu: In our lifetime*. London, England: Abacus.

South African History Online. (n.d.). *Albertina Nontsikelelo Sisulu*. Retrieved from http://www.sahistory.org.za/people

Wade, G. H., & Kasper, N. (2006). Nursing students' perceptions of instructor caring: An instrument based on Watson's theory of transpersonal caring. *Journal of Nursing Education, 45*(5), 162–168.

Watson, J. (1999). *Postmodern nursing and beyond*. Edinburgh, Scotland: Churchill Livingstone.

Watson, J. (2008). *Nursing: The philosophy and science of caring*. Boulder, CO: University Press of Colorado.

Whittemore, R., & Knafl, K. (2005). The integrative review: Updated methodology. *Journal of Advanced Nursing, 52*(5), 546–553.

CHAPTER FOURTEEN

# A Conceptual Framework for Midwifery in South Africa

*Anna Nolte*

### CARITAS QUOTE

*. . . and the only thing worth living for is love. Love for one another. Love for ourselves. Love for our work . . . . (Watson, 2013b, p. 262)*

*In this chapter, I describe my journey to Caring Science and Caritas. Then, I describe the three components of the Theory of Human Caring that resonate with me and my practice: the transpersonal relationship, the caring moment, and the Caritas Processes and how they relate to midwifery. Finally, I discuss how Dr. Watson's Theory of Human Caring and Ubuntu guide the practice of midwifery in South Africa.*

## ◼ OBJECTIVES

*The objectives of this chapter are to:*

- *Describe my personal journey with Caring Science and Caritas*
- *Describe key elements of Caring Science and Caritas relating to midwifery*
- *Describe how the theory will be implemented in my work—a conceptual framework for midwifery in South Africa*

## ■ JOURNEY TO CARING SCIENCE AND CARITAS

I am a midwife in South Africa and I was always interested in "caring," because that is what midwives should do. I developed some "caring standards" as part of a post-doctoral research in the late 1980s. When I decided to do a concept analysis of caring in midwifery, I came across the work of Dr. Jean Watson for the first time. It was a practical theory that could easily be applied in midwifery.

Life worked in wonderful miraculous ways for me to meet with Dr. Jean Watson during 2012 and 2014. First, Dr. Marie Hastings-Tolsma, a former faculty member at the University of Colorado in Denver, came to South Africa in 2011 as a Fulbright Scholar. We became friends and continued to communicate when she returned to the United States. I told her that I admired the work of Dr. Jean Watson. When I went to the United States in 2012 to visit her, she introduced me to Dr. Watson. That was one of the highlights in my career!

At the same time, somebody from South Africa attended a Caritas Coaching workshop in the United States and offered to host the International Caritas Conference in South Africa. Dr. Watson came to South Africa in early 2014 to explore the possibilities of holding the Caritas Conference in South Africa. Marie Hastings-Tolsma happened to be in South Africa at the same time and our paths crossed with Dr. Watson! I became involved in the planning and preparations of the Caritas Conference that was held in 2015 in Johannesburg, South Africa, another professional and personal highlight.

At about the same time, I also noted on the Caritas website information about a postdoctoral fellowship with Dr. Watson and immediately wrote her an e-mail. Another miracle happened at the same time; I was awarded a research grant to work on a "caring in midwifery" project, which enabled me to do the fellowship with Dr. Watson.

A colleague from South Africa, Charlenè Downing, and I attended our first intensive seminar, together with five other scholars in Boulder, Colorado, in July 2016. For me, it was a personal, as well as professional, retreat. It was an incredible experience to literally sit at the feet of such a formidable woman and to be enriched academically as well as personally. Not only does she have an awesome knowledge of philosophy, nursing, and her caring theory, but she is a living example of what she preaches! The loving-kindness that radiates from her is an encouragement for everybody around her "to also be a living example of caring."

The main purpose of my fellowship is not only to learn as much as possible from Dr. Watson regarding caring and to apply it to midwifery, but also to develop a "caring language for South Africa" within the Watson theory. There are many differences between the Western world and Africa, but also many similarities. This is also true for caring.

## ■ KEY ELEMENTS OF CARING SCIENCE AND CARITAS RELATING TO MIDWIFERY

The word *midwife* means "to be with women." The relationship between the midwife and the new mother and her family is paramount during the childbearing events.

The goal of nursing according to Watson (2012) is:

> . . . [T]o help people gain a higher degree of harmony that fosters self-knowledge, self-reverence, self-caring, self-control and self-healing processes . . . . The goal is pursued through the human-to-human caring process and spirit-to-spirit caring connections and relationship that respond to the subjective inner world of the person in such a way that the nurse/midwife helps individuals find meaning in their existence, disharmony, suffering and turmoil and promotes self-control, choice, self-knowledge and informed self-determination with health-illness decisions. (p. 61)

Various researchers have attempted to determine how women experienced their labor and identify their needs. This clearly resonates with the goal of nursing mentioned previously. The presence of the midwife and her relationship with each woman and family play an important role in midwifery caring, where the emphasis is mostly on issues other than sickness and suffering. This made me focus on the following Caritas aspects:

- The transpersonal relationship
- The caring moment
- The Caritas Processes

I have focused on the first Caritas Process as it is almost a prerequisite for the other caring processes to take place. If this is not present, the caring process cannot start.

## CARING MOMENT

The caring moment is when the midwife and person/persons come together in such a way that an occasion for human caring can happen. The occasion gives both an opportunity to decide how to be in the relationship and what to do with the moment (Watson, 2012). According to Sitzman and Watson (2014), the transpersonal caring moment transcends space and time like a pebble that causes ripples on a pond—it affects self and the other in widening circles. A caring moment involves an action of choice of both the nurse/midwife and the other. It gives both of them an opportunity to choose how to engage in the moment.

It may also allow for the presence of the spirit of both to be present. It conveys a concern for the inner lifeworld and personal meaning of each individual, who feels a connection with the other at the spirit level. It opens up possibilities for healing and human connection at a deeper level than physical interaction (Sitzman & Watson, 2014). It becomes *transpersonal caring*. It has the ability to expand the human capacities (Watson, 2012).

Both the cared-for and the caring person can be influenced by the caring moment through their choices and actions. The caregiver needs to be aware of her own consciousness and authentic presence of being in a caring moment. The values and views of the nurse are as relevant as those of the patient/client (Sitzman & Watson, 2014).

A transpersonal caring relationship is a special type of relationship where there is an intersubjective flow between the nurse/midwife and client. The nurse/midwife enters into the life space of the client and detects the other person's soul or spirit, and responds to the condition in such a way that the client has a release of subjective feelings and thoughts she had been longing to release. The compassionate nurse/midwife helps to put the client in the best position to access her own inner healing resources (Watson, 2012).

## CARITAS PROCESSES

The Caritas Processes form the basis for the caring relationship with the client. They reflect a deeper relationship based on love and caring.

*Caritas Process #1. Embrace altruistic values and practice loving-kindness with self and others* (Watson, 2008). Caring begins with being present and open to compassion, as well as expressing mercy, gentleness, loving-kindness, and equanimity toward and with self before one can offer compassionate caring to others.

> Loving kindness is not a style of behavior to be consistently modelled; it is an attitude, an intention, a stance . . . it is the will to love and care in whatever ways are meaningful and helpful within a given moment, within a given situation. (Sitzman & Watson, 2014, p. 45)

As a beginning, we have to learn how to offer caring, love, forgiveness, compassion, and mercy to ourselves before we can offer authentic caring and love to others. This is usually taught to the child and becomes more established with adulthood. It can be further facilitated through the exchange of attitudes and beliefs and of learning and role modeling that happens between the student nurse/midwife and the educator (Watson, 2013a). It further develops through personal experience and self-examination, as well as through relationships with other people. The process of self-discovery and mindfulness helps nurses/midwives to become aware of their own beliefs, values, and understanding.

Nurses/midwives often become worn down by trying to always care without attending to their own need for loving care. Nurses/midwives also have to be able to treat themselves with loving-kindness and equanimity, gentleness, and dignity before they can accept respect and care for others (Watson, 2008).

Different factors will influence the outward expression of caring and loving-kindness, while the inner resolve of the nurse/midwife to care and to love remains constant. Sitzman and Watson (2014) believe that many challenges can blunt the ability or desire for these values. Pondering, defining, and redefining these traits within the context of daily experience and evolving personal wisdom will help to keep altruism and loving-kindness fresh and personally meaningful. Sitzman and Watson (2014) suggest that the nurse/midwife should constantly practice and examine loving-kindness in herself and practice it with all she might encounter.

## ■ HOW THE THEORY WILL BE IMPLEMENTED IN MY WORK— A CONCEPTUAL FRAMEWORK FOR MIDWIFERY IN SOUTH AFRICA

There are very few conceptual models of caring in midwifery internationally. Different researchers have done meta-syntheses and qualitative research to determine how mothers experienced their labor and what their needs for caring were.

The importance of continuous presence of the midwife with women during labor has been emphasized in many research projects. Continuous presence of the midwife has been associated with an increase in the woman's sense of control and coping (Hodnett, Gates, Hofmeyr, Sakala, & Weston, 2011), has affected a woman's choice of pain relief (Hodnett et al., 2011; Howarth, Swain, & Treharne, 2011), and is important for maternal–child attachment and the well-being of the new family (Howarth et al., 2011). It is proposed that midwives, who work "with" women in labor, experience a greater job satisfaction and are more likely to find their work emotionally rewarding (Hunter, 2004). In a study by Thelin, Lundgren, and Hermansson (2014), the authors found that it was important for midwives to be intentionally and authentically present as much as they could. The results from this study also showed that the midwives were empowered by the responses from the women and their partners. This empowerment was important for the individual midwife, her process of growth, and her self-confidence in being a midwife.

Halldorsdottir and Karlsdottir (1996) described the experience of women during the birth process. Results revealed an overarching theme encompassing the women's perceptions of caring and uncaring. This theme was identified as empowerment or discouragement. Two categories were identified within empowerment. In the first category, the midwife was perceived as caring and was seen as an indispensable presence throughout the delivery process. In the second category, emphasis was placed on the client's sense of empowerment. They (Halldorsdottir & Karlsdottir, 1996) described empowerment when the midwife strengthens the woman's confidence, facilitating recognition of her own strengths and capacities. The next two categories, where the midwife was perceived as uncaring, were consistent with the biocidic or life-destroying mode in Halldorsdottir's (1991) theory. These uncaring behaviors led the women to feel discouraged.

Matthews and Callister (2004) found that women experienced encouragement, continuity of care, knowledge, and dignity from midwives. Lundgren and

Berg (2007), in a meta-synthesis of eight qualitative studies, identified six pairs of concepts that are essential for the midwife–woman relationship. It is essential to meet and respond to the childbearing woman's surrendering, trust, participation, loneliness, difference, and creation of meaning. The midwife's response should include availability, mediation of trust, mutuality, and confirmation, as well as support uniqueness and meaningfulness. Berg (2005) identified that a dignity-protective relationship is an essential component of midwifery care for pregnant women. Five overlapping elements were included, namely mutuality, trust, ongoing dialogue, shared responsibilities, and enduring presence.

In another synthesis of qualitative studies, Bowers (2002) found that women expect to be supported through their physical comfort. They also expect emotional support through presence, encouragement, and communication with a caring tone. Most women want to be included in the decision-making process. Laboring women expect that the midwife will have the necessary knowledge and experience.

Midwives' uncaring behaviors as perceived by women have also been described. For example, women have felt ignored when midwives did not speak to them or give updated information (Eliasson, Kainz, & von Post, 2008). The mothers could also not attract a midwife's attention, causing mothers to feel mistrust. Physical uncaring acts were also perceived by women who experienced careless physical care in which the mothers' sense of dignity was offended and humiliated. Lack of empathy, spiritual presence, and kindness on the part of midwives caused mothers to be traumatized and disempowered, sometimes reliving their distress long after birth (Moloney & Gair, 2015).

## ■ MIDWIFERY IN SOUTH AFRICA

Midwifery care in our country experiences many challenges at present; for example, the maternal mortality rate is still very high. Midwives are involved in an increasing number of medical-legal cases. The complaints involved include negligence, sexual assault, a lack of skills, system failures, and other errors. A shortage of midwives and a lack of adequate facilities and other resources cause midwives to end up drained, exhausted, and struggling to cope with the overwhelming workload.

In our research to determine midwives' experience of practicing midwifery in South Africa, we learned that midwives agreed that there is a great shortage of midwives in South Africa, which is worse in public than private hospitals (Hastings-Tolsma & Nolte, 2014). The high numbers of births in public hospitals make the situation worse. The fact that midwives are so busy contributes to midwives being unable to give individual attention and support to mothers, forcing them to leave mothers alone for long periods of time. The midwives reported,

> . . . *because of workload, staff shortages, yes, you cannot give them your entire support and care.*

*Two professional midwives working at day shift . . . and we are very busy—sometimes more than 20 births.*

*There just isn't time . . . you literally run from bed to bed catching babies.*

This workload caused midwives to become exhausted.

*Sometimes you feel that you work without a break, without lunch, without tea and by the time you go home, you can't even eat or wash, that is how exhausted you are.*

The lack of physical resources is a further burden for midwives to function effectively. Midwives who worked public hospitals complained about their lack of resources.

*Some patients bring their own bedding and sheets . . . in addition to their own pads and we appreciate that.*

It is not always possible for mothers to have somebody with them during labor, because of a lack of space in the labor wards and concerns about security. Privacy is also a problem, because many labor wards are open wards.

*. . . . it is not allowed, there is no space . . . here is one bed this side the other bed this side . . . so there can be no privacy.*

*. . . we do not allow it because it's an open setting and we look at the dignity of the patient so we don't allow, we protect the other patients who have got a low threshold to pain because they undress and cry and vomit and so on . . .*

This means that if midwives were not present, most women were totally without support during labor.

The large numbers of patients seem to be a big burden on the already existing shortage of midwives and resources.

*You continuously take in patients whether the hospital is full whether there is no space.*

Midwives are often being accused of being disrespectful to patients and they are aware of this image.

*. . . public find midwives very abusive—because they smack them.*

Many patients do not want to deliver in hospitals . . . *because they are frightened of midwives.*

Another reason for the harsh behavior is the perception that midwives do not have a passion to care:

*Many midwives train to be one because it is a job . . . they have no passion or desire to care for people . . . that is what is creating the problem for how the public sees midwives. . . .*

This study has provided some insight about what midwives experience as important factors that have an influence on their relationship and caring of child-bearing women.

Halldorsdottir (1991) developed a continuum from uncaring to caring. Uncaring can be classified as biocidic, which can be life destroying, leading to anger, despair, and decreased well-being. Biostatic is life restraining; the patient experienced the nurse as cold and treatment as a nuisance. Biopassive is life neutral; the nurse is apathetic and detached.

Caring can be classified as bioactive—it is life sustaining. The nurse is viewed as kind and concerned. Biogenic is the highest level of human-to-human caring; it is life giving and life receiving for both nurse and patient. It seems as if the caring in the previous research (Hastings-Tolsma & Nolte, 2014) can be classified as biocidic and biostatic.

The following possible solutions to this problem will be explored, namely to use Watson's philosophy and theory as a conceptual framework for midwifery in South Africa. The following priorities were determined to start this process, namely:

- To look at the Watson theory through an African lens and an African ontology, namely Ubuntu, and to compare the values and ethics of Ubuntu with that of the Watson theory
- To determine how midwives in South Africa can internalize the first carative process in order to enable them to offer compassionate caring to others

## WATSON'S THEORY IN MIDWIFERY

Watson's theory is a nursing theory. One of the main differences between nursing and midwifery is that pregnancy and childbearing is mostly a physiological process and not illness, like in many nursing cases. Watson's definition of caring (see Part Two) makes as much provision for healthy clients as for sick patients. Watson's value system consists of values associated with deep respect for the wonders and mysteries of life and acknowledgment of a spiritual dimension to life and internal power of the human caring process, growth, and change, which is so important in midwifery. Emphasis is placed on helping a person gain more self-knowledge, self-control, self-caring, and inner healing of self. This resonates with the women's experiences and needs as described earlier.

The first carative process will be as important in midwifery as in nursing. The midwife will have to practice loving-kindness/compassion and equanimity with self /other. This will serve as a prerequisite for all the other carative processes to follow. All the carative factors will fit and should be applied in the midwifery process. In the caring moment like in nursing, the occasion involves action and choice by both the individual and the midwife, which leads to the decision on how to be in the relationship—what to do with the moment.

## UBUNTU

Ubuntu is indigenous to Africa. Many sub-Saharan languages have versions of the word *Ubuntu* in their respective languages. It is difficult to translate into English; however, it roughly means "humanness" or "a person is a person through other persons." It is seen as a tradition—from parents and tribal practices inherited from the past. It is also seen as moral values and indigenous culture codes. Some described it as sanctioned by gods and ancestors. Some authors described it as a fundamental ontology and epistemological category in African thought. The concept was first used as a postamble in the interim constitution of South Africa in 1993:

> There is a need for understanding, but not for vengeance, a need for reparation, but not for retaliation, a need for Ubuntu, but not for victimization. (Constitution of the Republic of South Africa, Act 200 of 1993, in Gade, 2011)

The new government of South Africa in 1994 adopted Ubuntu as a concept to foster a stronger sense of unity. The policy of Ubuntu is explained in the White Paper where it was used as a principle of "caring of each other's well-being . . . , respect for human rights and responsibilities in promoting well-being of the individuals and societal well-being" (Mbaya, 2010, p. 373).

The main attribute of Ubuntu is a *deep rootedness in community*. Identities are formed through the community: A person is who he is because of the existence and relationship with/of others and because of coexistence with them. There is a combination of mainly two forms of interaction—identity (sharing a way of life) and solidarity—(caring for others—quality of life).

The other attributes in short are as follows:

- *Respect and dignity.* It acknowledges the rights and responsibilities of every citizen. Every other person is seen as oneself and should be treated with respect. Others' needs are met at equal measure as one's own.
- *Solidarity* is demonstrated through mutual responsibility and recognition. Survival comes through a collective and collaborative spirit.
- *Spirituality* lies in a person's connection to other people and the universe; a strong personal faith drives you.
- *Reciprocity.* Relations involve exchange.
- *Harmony* and group cohesion and agreement are strong concepts. It is created through trust, fairness, and shared understanding. One does not feel threatened by others.
- *Mutuality* is a touchstone—mutual trust, caring, support, responsibility, and recognition. Relations are paramount. People are bound together in an ethic of care and respect.
- *Affinity and kinship.* The following concepts demonstrate affinity and caring: compassion, at center, humanness—the essence of being a person, kindness, care, loving-kindness, acceptance, empathy, friendliness, and helpfulness.

(Beets, 2012; Bell & Metz, 2011; Chinouya & O'Keefe, 2006; Dolamo, 2013; Metz & Gaie, 2010; Murithi, 2006; Prinsloo, 2001; van der Walt, 2010).

## ■ CONCLUSION

The next task during the postdoctoral scholarship will be to do a thorough comparison of Watson's theory and Ubuntu. It appears superficially as if there are many commonalities. Both are based on an intentionality to care for the other person, which is based on loving-kindness and compassion.

## ■ REFERENCES

Beets, P. A. D. (2012). Strengthening morality and ethics in educational assessment through Ubuntu in South Africa. *Educational Philosophy and Theory, 44*(S2), 68–83.

Bell, D. A., & Metz, T. (2011). Confucianism and Ubuntu: Reflections on a dialogue between Chinese and African traditions. *Journal of Chinese Philosophy, 38*(Suppl.), 78–95.

Berg, M. (2005). A midwifery model of care for childbearing women at high risk: Genuine caring in caring for the genuine. *Journal of Perinatal Education, 14*, 9–21.

Bowers, B. B. (2002). Mother's experience of labor support: Exploration of qualitative research. *Journal of Obstetric, Gynecologic, and Neonatal Nursing, 31*, 742–752.

Chinouya, M., & O'Keefe, E. (2006). Zimbabwean cultural traditions in England: Ubuntu-Hunhu as a human rights tool. *Diversity in Health and Social Care, 3*, 89–98.

Dolamo, R. (2013). Botho/Ubuntu: The heart of African ethics. *Scriptura, 112*, 1–10.

Eliasson, M., Kainz, G., & von Post, I. (2008). Uncaring midwives. *Nursing Ethics, 15*, 500–511.

Gade, C. B. N. (2011). The historical development of the written discourses on Ubuntu. *South African Journal Philosophy, 30*, 303–329.

Halldorsdottir, S. (1991). Five basic modes of being with another. In D. A. Gaut & M. M. Leininger (Eds.), *Caring: The compassionate healer* (pp. 37–49). New York, NY: National League for Nursing.

Halldorsdottir, S., & Karlsdottir, S. I. (1996). Empowerment or discouragement: Women's experience of caring and uncaring encounters during childbirth. *Health Care International, 17*, 361–379.

Hastings-Tolsma, M., & Nolte, A. G. W. (2014, June). Birth stories of women and midwives in South Africa. Paper presented at the 30th Triennial International Congress of Midwives, Prague, Czech Republic.

Hodnett, E. D., Gates, S., Hofmeyr, G. J., Sakala, C., & Weston, J. (2011). Continuous support for women during childbirth. *Cochrane Database of Systematic Reviews, 2*, CD003766.

Howarth, H., Swain, N., & Treharne, G. J. (2011). First-time New Zealand mothers' experience of birth: Importance of relationship and support. *New Zealand College of Midwives Journal, 45*, 6–11.

Hunter, B. (2004). Conflicting ideologies as a source of emotion work in midwifery. *Midwifery, 20*, 261–272.

Lundgren, I., & Berg, M. (2007). Central concepts in the midwife-woman relationship. *Scandinavian Journal of Caring Science, 21*, 220–228.

Matthews, R., & Callister, L. C. (2004). Childbearing women's perceptions of nursing care that promotes dignity. *Journal of Obstetric, Gynecologic, and Neonatal Nursing, 33*, 498–507.

Mbaya, H. (2010). Social capital and the imperatives of the concept and life of Ubuntu in the South African context. *Scriptura, 104*, 367–376.

Metz, T., & Gaie, B. R. (2010). The African ethic of Ubuntu/Botho: Implications for research on morality. *Journal of Moral Education, 39*(3), 273–290.

Moloney, S., & Gair, S. (2015). Empathy and spiritual care in midwifery practice: Contributing to women's enhanced birth experiences. *Women and Birth, 28*(4), 323–328. doi:10.1016/j.wombi .2015.04.009

Murithi, T. (2006). Practical peacemaking wisdom for Africa: Reflections on Ubuntu. *Journal of Pan African Studies, 1*(4), 25–34.

Prinsloo, E. D. (2001). A comparison between medicine from an African (Ubuntu) and Western philosophy. *Curationis, 24*, 58–65. doi:10.4102/curationis.v24i1.802

Sitzman, K., & Watson, J. (2014). *Caring science, mindful practice: Implementing Watson's human caring theory.* New York, NY: Springer Publishing.

Thelin, I. L., Lundgren, I., & Hermansson, E. (2014). Midwives' lived experience of caring during childbearing—A phenomenological study. *Sexual & Reproductive Healthcare, 5*, 113–118.

van der Walt, J. L. (2010). Ubuntu waardes: Samelewings en pedagogiese verwagtinge. *Tydskrif vir Geesteswetenskappe, 50*(2), 229–242.

Watson, J. (2008). *Nursing. The philosophy and science of caring* (Rev. ed.). Boulder, CO: University Press of Colorado.

Watson, J. (2012). *Human caring science* (2nd ed.). Sudbury, MA: Jones & Bartlett.

Watson, J. (2013a). Nursing: The philosophy and science of caring. In M. C. Smith, M. C. Turkel, & Z. R. Wolf (Eds.), *Caring in nursing classics: An essential resource* (pp. 143–153). New York, NY: Springer Publishing.

Watson, J. (2013b). Nursing: The philosophy and science of caring (Rev. ed.). In M. C. Smith, M. C. Turkel, & Z. R. Wolf (Eds.), *Caring in nursing classics: An essential resource* (pp. 243–263). New York, NY: Springer Publishing.

# CHAPTER FIFTEEN

# Caritas for Society's Safe-Keepers: Upholding Human Dignity and Caring

Joseph Giovannoni

---

### CARITAS QUOTE

*Sustaining humanistic-altruistic values by practice of loving-kindness compassion, and equanimity with self/other. (Watson, n.d., Caritas Process #1)*

---

*For the past 35 years as a forensic advanced practice nurse, I have worked to rehabilitate patients who are adjudicated sex offenders, drug abusers, and domestic violence abusers. My work is guided by the legal system. However, the work is largely an interprofessional collaboration. Interprofessional collaboration requires joint commitment and mutual trust, since rehabilitation requires patients to waive their confidentiality to ensure community safety. The professionals working jointly with me are Society's Safe-Keepers, people who can bring the light of caring to those who engage in darkness.*

## ■ OBJECTIVES

*The objectives of this chapter are to:*

• *Describe the contemporary application of Caring Science to rehabilitation science and judicial system operations*

- *Define the role and responsibilities of the Society's Safe-Keepers*
- *Discuss the strategies to rehabilitate violent offenders with Caritas*
- *Understand the role of the Caritas as a therapeutic process to heal both the parole officer and the perpetrator*

Society's Safe-Keepers[1] (SSKs) embrace compassion and human dignity while implementing evidence-based, or informed (DiNapoli, Turkel, Nelson, & Watson, 2010) practices, in order to be positive caring role models for their patients, those who have behaved uncaringly toward others. SSKs are professionals dedicated to protecting society by rehabilitating others. I created the name SSK to describe my interdisciplinary team. SSKs are not administrators of punishment; instead, they believe in justice and human dignity, and promote faith, hope, and peace in our society. SSKs are responsible for rehabilitating individuals who have violated the rights and human dignity of others. SSKs are trained to correct cognitive distortions and the core beliefs that justified past acts of violence and the exploitation of others. They are conscious that change, or rehabilitation, can only occur in a transpersonal caring relationship. They believe that protecting society from tyranny requires a philosophy of caring and respect for all of humanity. This chapter describes SSKs and how they are successful in rehabilitating adjudicated sex offenders, substance abusers, and perpetrators of domestic violence.

Who are the SSKs? These professionals include probation/parole officers, as well as forensic professionals such as psychiatric mental health nurses, psychiatrists, social workers, psychologists, forensic counselors, and law enforcers. An important role of the SSK is to collaborate with all interested parties in using combined wisdom to prevent violence. They choose this profession to help others find positive prosocial means to cope. The competence of an SSK is proportional to the SSK's courage to explore, acknowledge, and address his or her own wounding, and to revisit the validity of long-held beliefs and prejudices (Giovannoni, 2016). They must be self-aware of their motives, practice self-care, and remain nonjudgmental. These compassionate professionals may gravitate to this work because they also need personal healing.

## ■ SSKs: ROLE MODELS OF LOVE AND COMPASSION?

My patients represent different ethnicities with various socioeconomic statuses. The patients who are laborers or homeless come to my office sweaty, dirty, and exhausted. Colleagues who witness my work believe my practice assimilates a mission of love and compassion. The humanity I treat refutes the power of the light

---

[1] Society's Safe-Keepers © 2013 Joseph Giovannoni.

of the loving consciousness within them and are driven by fear and darkness. Their offenses reflect a need for immediate gratification to cope with their fears and sense of lacking control. These patients have no concern for the victim(s) they target. They function from a primitive consciousness, what neuroscientists refer to as the reptile brain, the limbic system (Linden, 2011). They are informed by core beliefs such as "no one tells me what to do."

The patients often make excuses, while some turn to religion for forgiveness. In the absolution of forgiveness, the patients believe they are not responsible for making restitution to their victim(s). They also rationalize their behavior: "I am a sinner . . . we are all sinners." In the case of the sex offender, they blame the child for sexually provoking them. They lack balance between the forces of human desire that originate in the brain's limbic system to sustain their human needs and a consciousness that reflects compassion for self and others. Similar to our early ancestors who lived in caves, these violent offenders operate out of fear, the instinct for survival, the need for self-gratification, and the desire for external power.

Although I am painting a dark picture of the humanity I treat, we all possess a dark side. In statements such as "I hate you," the dark side surfaces. Understanding the early evolution of the dark side is important, as most of my patients have a history of dysfunctional family dynamics, have experienced neglect, are emotionally detached, and have adjustment disorders. SSKs are forensic professionals engaged in the enlightened rehabilitation practices, cognizant of the power of the compassionate heart and the practice of loving-kindness in transforming those who have behaved in an unloving way. A compassionate intention is a modeling method functioning as a catalyst to light compassion in others who are stuck in darkness. Modeling compassion and loving-kindness teaches the development of a concern for others.

In my work, I have helped patients with antisocial personality and psychopathy progress to become authentically compassionate human beings. These transformations require SSKs to hold patients accountable for their actions with loving-kindness. Professionals who embrace the powers of their intelligent heart intuitively are present and authentic, and set limits with a kind demeanor. Role models acting in loving-kindness teach others how to better meet their own needs without exploiting others. Those SSKs who authentically arm themselves with the power of their compassionate heart are more likely to influence others to respect and share humanity.

## ■ SELF-CARE FOR SSKs: LOVING-KINDNESS FOR SELF

In order to maintain equanimity and effectively extend help to others, SSKs must practice loving-kindness and compassion for self (Giovannoni, McCoy, Mays, & Watson, 2015; Watson, 2008). SSKs must explore painful experiences that inform their lives and understand how job-related stress can trigger symptoms that may cause the revisiting of past personal trauma. Self-compassion and self-care are essential for them to authentically extend loving-kindness to others. Compassion for self begins by understanding the complexity of cause and effect in our world. We need to consciously let go of the past and be mindful that we are no longer victims of past experiences (Hawkins, 2012). Personally, my equanimity is sustained by heart-centered breathing, consciously breathing in love, and breathing out to release the past.

As an SSK leader, my professional life is dedicated to understanding the causes of violence. For this, I turn to science, but I find that science is not sufficient. Instead, I choose to see my patients as my teachers. For the patient to become my teacher, I need to be present in the moment, observe the behavior, and understand the patient's history without engaging in judgment. We cannot overlook the lack of consciousness of the unity of the mind as a contributor to the absence of compassion for others. The ego-centered core beliefs that separate us from others, together with personal prejudices, create a strong barrier of judgment. This judgment prevents the mind from experiencing compassion for self and others. To maintain equanimity—minimal stress with keen objectivity—we need to be mindful in letting go. Without this, SSKs are vulnerable to project countertransference onto those they are entrusted to help. If SSKs do not resolve their own past trauma and prejudices, they are vulnerable to abusing their power and punishing the patient.

Among SSKs, job-related stress can lead to poor performance and high staff turnover (Simmons, Cochran, & Blount, 1997). Stress and burnout result when employees feel devalued (Brown, 1987; Risdon, Wells, & Wesley, 2003). SSKs read many victim statements containing detailed descriptions of the victims' trauma. Vicarious trauma can occur when we are repeatedly exposed to traumatized victims or the details of traumatic experiences (McCann & Pearlman, 1990). In an effort to cope, some SSKs emotionally engage in self-protection by becoming distant and cold. This results in detached interactions, where others are treated as a nuisance.

In helping professions, burnout occurs when helpers become uncaring (Watson, 2008). A lack of caring, added to frustration and anger, can lead to SSKs objectifying their patients. An emotionally detached and uncaring professional mirrors the same uncaring objectification his or her patient engaged in with their victim(s). The SSK must practice self-care to heal past traumas. In this attempt to avoid vicarious trauma, the SSK needs to avoid suppressing his or her feelings. When we operate out of fear, we often create illusory self-protective boundaries. Monitoring our thoughts and feelings in interactions with patients and colleagues is essential for maintaining mental equilibrium. We need to develop a program of self-care to prevent stress that leads to burnout.

The practice of loving-kindness, compassion, and equanimity with self and others reduces stress and facilitates an authentic presence (Giovannoni, McCoy, Mays, & Watson, 2015). When we recognize the encroachment of judgment and the feeling of being overwhelmed, practicing self-compassion and self-forgiveness is a healthy self-initiated therapy. Forgiveness is often misunderstood; it does not excuse uncaring behaviors. True forgiveness is a process of relinquishing grievances because they serve no purpose, rather than inflict self-imposed suffering and pain. Forgiveness is correcting the thoughts and core beliefs that our ego embraces to justify hurting and exploiting strangers, as well as our colleagues, friends, and family.

## ■ FROM EGO'S DIVIDED PERCEPTION TO UNITY OF MIND

The ego-personality is informed by the five senses (Zukav, 2014). When the senses are not working in tandem, we are vulnerable to experiencing a divided self that is motivated by fear and the need for survival. The ego perception of separateness is a source of fear that can trigger anger and that is the barrier to peace. A violent personality operates from the ego-divided consciousness and hurts others because the ego-self feels powerless. The ego-centered personality seeks external power by preying on others. From 30 years of forensic work, my anecdotal observation is that the ego's attempt to compensate for feelings of powerlessness is the core contributor to violence. This situation can also result between colleagues who operate out of personal ego-agendas in an attempt to control others.

## ■ CARING SCIENCE

Human consciousness is an innate desire to awaken to the creative power of the vision of oneness the presence that extends concern and compassion for self and others. This is the essence of humanity, the desire for spiritual awakening. Spirituality evolves by the repeated practice of acting out of concern for others. A renaissance of compassion, caring, and love has emerged in the health sciences (Watson, 2008). Dr. Jean Watson's Caring Science is well developed, often practiced, and validated through studies in health care sciences. This science can also be integrated into forensic science. Caring Science takes the perspective that humanity resides in a unitary or undivided field of consciousness (Levinas, 2000[1969]; Levinas, Poller, & Cohen, 2003; Watson, 2008). In its wisdom, Caring Science encourages us to return to compassion, caring, and universal love—the authentic power necessary to develop transpersonal caring relationships. Practicing and embodying this unitary theoretical model facilitated balance in my personal and professional lives. Beyond the darkness of the separated ego's structure, wholeness of mind resides still. The mind is universal and connected to the source, or the omniscience, omnipotence, and omnipresence of love. The mind is the creative self that has advanced humanity toward compassion and unity. The ego is the self that identifies with the body and utilizes the five senses to program the brain to respond in survival mode. The ego is separate and cannot conceive wholeness or unity. Instead, the ego focuses on its own agendas and desires external power. Authentic internal power can only evolve when we create a balance between the ego-personality and a consciousness of unity.

Dr. Watson often reminds us that we are "one mind and one heart." This profound statement shifts our consciousness, as well as proposes the solution to violence. Unity of the mind, the relationship between compassion, love, and justice, needs to be understood and embraced. Chaos in society cannot be corrected by force but rather by a life-giving philosophy that unites humanity. Compassionate universalism bridges separation and reminds us to shift from a perception of duality, separation, and ego-centeredness to a vision of oneness. From the source, we can begin to develop and sustain loving and trusting relationships (Ray, 2010). Compassion heals our whole human family. The focus on human differences such as race, gender, economic status, nationalism, and religion perpetuates discord, and the love of external power obstructs authentic spiritual development. The result is conflict. The love of power reflects a mind that is conflicted and divided. Self-centered, absorbed by power, and limited to the input provided by our sensory systems, the ego's primary goal is immediate gratification. A lack of concern for others inhibits the evolution of the human spirit. In my practice, I observed this lack of concern in sex offenders and violent individuals. The source of their wrongful behavior was the expression of their ego's sense of emptiness, their lack of self-compassion, their fears, and their need to compensate by overpowering another. Mahatma Gandhi stated, "The day the power of love overrules the love of power, the world will know peace" (Alli, 2013, p. 34).

## ■ MORAL AND ETHICAL OBLIGATIONS

The patients I treat are lost in darkness as they operate from their primitive selfish ego. They cope with an emotionally detached sense of self by engaging in thrill-seeking sexual behavior and mood-altering drugs. When their behavior hurts another person, they refuse to accept responsibility. Hidden from their consciousness is the seed of compassion, and authentic love for self remains dormant. The dormancy is the condition requiring treatment. Rarely do patients in this population voluntarily seek help. I frequently listen to horrific stories of sexual violence; these stories can make SSKs angry, cynical, and fearful, and trigger a sense of being devalued when help is not accepted. These are the symptoms of vicarious trauma (McCann & Pearlman, 1990). Sex offenders are often manipulative and resentful, and behave passive aggressively and disrespectfully. They are court-ordered into treatment and they displace their resentment onto SSKs. Despite this, SSKs cannot risk becoming unkind. SSKs must be careful not to displace the negativity absorbed from negative interactions onto patients, colleagues, or their families.

Given this scenario, we understand why some people hold a fatalistic sentiment toward this population and are pejorative about rehabilitation. Commonly, people ask, "Why bother treating these individuals?" Newscasters and the public refer to sex offenders as "monsters." This collective ego, a fearful mentality, is focused on the problem rather than on developing creative solutions. As SSKs, we are vigilant so that we do not become discouraged. We need to educate society as to the cause of humanity's darkness. Our society has a moral and ethical obligation to educate and rehabilitate these individuals. Locking them up and throwing away the proverbial key, as some suggest, reflects thinking from the dark ages. Our society needs to understand the cause of sexual violence and how the perception of duality contributes. Forensic science must rapidly mature to embrace the philosophy of unity and compassion as the treatment for maladaptive antisocial behavior.

Patients come from all walks of life. They are often legitimate and even respected members of the community. Much of my work can be mechanical. My practice requires addressing the "dynamic risk factors" of sex offending behavior and applying informed interventions such as cognitive behavioral therapy to address the risk and the offender's needs (Andrews, Zinger, Hoge, Gendreau, & Cullen, 2006). I am neither required nor mandated to integrate human caring and compassion into my practice. Importantly, I have not come across discussions in the literature specific to incorporating compassion into the treatment of such offenders. However, the peer-reviewed literature is sparse in providing solutions. Promoting treatment as an option for some offenders over long-term incarceration is seen as bureaucratic compassion. However, treating rather than punishing the offender is cost-effective for society and proven to be more effective for patients assessed to be at low risk of re-offending (Prescott & Levenson, 2010).

## ■ INTEGRATING CARING SCIENCE WITH FORENSIC SCIENCE—A CONUNDRUM?

We can no longer disregard the value of integrating compassion as a therapeutic solution to prevent violence. A caring approach while holding perpetrators accountable may be viewed as a contradictory conundrum. Traditionally, violence is a problem addressed with punishment. The relevance of human caring is not discussed in the scientific tradition. Motivational interviewing to facilitate cooperation to change behavior seems sufficient and its efficacy has been documented (Miller & Rollnick, 2002). The "Good Lives" model and positive psychology are comprehensive approaches that have emerged in the treatment of sex offenders (Ward & Gannon, 2006; Wong, 2011). These approaches focus on teaching positive interactions and facilitate virtue, resilience, and well-being. High-energy powerful words with related actions, such as compassion and loving-kindness, are necessary to shape good lives that include a genuine concern for the well-being of others.

How do we support our patients in developing concern for others, if we are not authentic role models of human caring? Society's contemporary sentiment is to be hard on criminals; however, this ideology *has not* decreased crime. As such, we need to consider creative early interventions in the development of a child, which include fostering caring relationships within the family. Most of my patients have a history of family dysfunction and abandonment. Fostering human caring has to have priority over academic competition in educational systems. An environment of loving-kindness must also be nurtured in the penal system if we are to rehabilitate inmates to care for themselves and for others. Attempting to rehabilitate the criminal mind without compassion can harden our hearts, contribute to stress, and create negative relationships. If we are to eradicate violence, we must consider the power of authentic loving-kindness to correct the beliefs that justify violating human rights. Compassionate interactions are life giving (Watson, 2008). Forensic bureaucracy cannot deny that violence reflects a lack of compassion and caring for others. We have a responsibility to be role models of compassion if we are to develop a compassionate society. Love prevails over fear and neutralizes the ego's desire for the external power responsible for criminal behavior. Removing a dangerous criminal perpetrator from the community into confinement may be necessary in some situations and is an act of caring to protect society. Any confinement to rehabilitate an inmate needs to be in a healing environment focused on caring and maintaining human dignity. A prison system devoid of human caring is neither "correctional" nor "rehabilitative." The professionals working daily with the criminal population acknowledge the work is emotional and stressful. Over the years I have witnessed substantial staff turnover attributable to burnout. Burnout can be prevented through the protective resilience resulting from practicing compassion and loving-kindness toward self.

Caring Science provides mindful practices such as embracing "cultivating the practice of loving-kindness and equanimity toward self and others" (Watson, 2008). We can learn how to be authentically present without judgment. We can be inspired to be hopeful and to honor others. We can center and be mindful as we listen to another person's story while accepting and acknowledging our positive and negative feelings. We can nurture trusting and caring relationships. Caring Science informs cognitive behavioral therapy by nurturing beliefs to enhance personal growth and better practices. Balance is established by addressing individual needs and recognizing readiness for change. Our practice is deepened by focusing on creative solutions and innovative methods for caring decision making.

## ■ FOCUSING ON SOLUTIONS AND NOT ON THE PROBLEM

From my extensive SSK experience, I believe violence results when a person separates from his or her humanity and treats others as objects. This results when the ego's personal agendas are dominant, disavowing the presence of a higher self that connects all humanity with the infinite source of love. The solution to stemming violence is to practice and teach the unitary belief that we are all connected to the infinite source, and to promote the belief in justice, equality, human dignity, and the covenant to honor the human spirit. Caring Science offers a unitary worldview based on the philosophy and ethic of *belonging*, in that everything in the universe is connected and *belongs* to the infinite oneness of all (Levinas, 2000[1969]; Watson, 2005, 2008). Embodying this consciousness embraces the safety of humanity.

In the treatment of sex abusers, SSKs must adhere to the best rehabilitative practices (Andrews et al., 2006) and the code of ethics guidelines of the Association for the Treatment of Sexual Abusers (ATSA). A mechanical application of evidence-based interventions and motivational interviewing without the intention of authentic compassion may suffice for some; however, this may result in a disingenuous therapist. Informed by a unitary theory and embodying loving-kindness and compassion, I facilitate cooperative relationships. SSKs with a caring intentionality are intuitive, remain vigilant, and observe and discern without being threatening, enhancing patient motivation. This is the SSK, praxis, or the "informed practice; practice that is empirically validated and informed by one's philosophical-ethical-theoretical orientation, but grounded in concrete actions and behaviors that can be empirically assessed and measured" (DiNapoli et al., 2010, p. 16).

By practicing Caring Science, I can be peaceful, compassionate, and loving as I administer scientific interventions. Working toward a solution to violence requires authentic, compassionate, and caring professionals. By extending caring to those who have behaved unlovingly toward others, we are not creating a contradiction in therapy. Instead, we need to clarify what it means to be loving and compassionate. Watson (2008) connects love with the Latin word *Caritas*, which denotes "caring or love for something that lies beyond the self-interest of any given individual" (p. 253). Caritas represents compassion and generosity of spirit.

The ego perception of separation focuses on self-interest and disregards compassion. This dark quality in humanity is founded in fear and the need for survival. A lack of Caritas is the fundamental cause of the exploitation of others. Seeing oneself as separate from another is a barrier to human compassion. We are, however, part of the same cosmic fabric. Forensic professionals in the criminal justice system are vulnerable to raising barriers that reflect negative corrosive interactions. These interactions can occur with patients but also with colleagues. If we close our heart, we can easily become frustrated, stressed, and void of human dignity. When we practice Caritas, we become role models for compassion who radiate an energetic healing environment (Watson, 2008).

Building safer communities is not accomplished without compassion. Violence is not resolved by focusing on the problem. Resolution emerges from understanding the nature of our being and the practice of Caritas. A vision for a healthier and safer community *cannot* be achieved with an ideology of punishment. Informed practices and interventions, administered with compassion, caring, and loving-kindness, are the solution. Compassionate universalism requires all aspects of humanity—political, institutional, social, cultural, and criminal justice—to be guided by compassion to solve the problem of violence. Ray (2010) argues, "the new ethics of compassion, patient rights, cultural rights, and cultural justice will become central to understanding morally right action in choice making." SSKs must not forget that the authentic power of their compassionate heart is a solution to violence.

## ■ CONCLUSION

Those who treat violent offenders cannot afford to close their hearts by becoming emotionally detached. When SSKs practice without caring, love, and compassion, they create cold, mechanical interactions. Role models of caring are needed to rehabilitate perpetrators who have harmed others. Cold and judgmental interactions will not teach patients how to be respectful and caring. Accepting responsibility and being accountable for actions is fundamental to caring. A role model of human caring is a necessary catalyst to motivate patients to develop empathy and to make restitution to those they harmed. Energetic, authentic, caring SSKs observe and discern, sustain human dignity, and do not judge. They create cooperative healing environments by cultivating the practice of loving-kindness with self and others. They nurture transpersonal life-giving interactions as they apply informed practices and interventions: the SSK praxis.

## ■ REFERENCES

Alli, I. (2013). *101 selected sayings of Mahatma Gandhi.* Sudbury, MA: eBookIt.

Andrews, D., Zinger, I., Hoge, R. D., Gendreau, P., & Cullen, F. (2006). Does correctional treatment work? A clinically relevant and psychologically informed meta-analysis. *Criminology, 28*(3), 369–404. doi:10.1111/j.1745–9125.1990.tb01330.x

Brown, P. W. (1987). Probation officer burnout: An organizational disease/an organizational cure. *Federal Probation, 51*(3), 17–21. Retrieved from https://www.ncjrs.gov/pdffiles1/Digitization/108633NCJRS.pdf

DiNapoli, P. P., Turkel, M., Nelson, J., & Watson, J. (2010). Measuring the Caritas processes: Caring factor survey. *International Journal for Human Caring, 14*(3), 15–20.

Giovannoni, J. (2016). Egoless and interconnected: Suspending judgment to embrace heart-centered health care. In W. Rosa (Ed.), *Nurses as leaders: Evolutionary visions of leadership* (Chapter 19). New York, NY: Springer Publishing.

Giovannoni, J., McCoy, K. T., Mays, M., & Watson, J. (2015). Probation officers reduce their stress by cultivating the practice of loving-kindness with self and others. *International Journal of Caring Sciences, 8*(2), 325–343.

Hawkins, D. (2012). *Letting go: The pathway of surrender.* New York, NY: Hay House.

Levinas, E. (2000[1969]). *Totality and infinity.* Pittsburgh, PA: Duquesne.

Levinas, E., Poller, N., & Cohen, R. (2003). *Humanism of the other.* Chicago, IL: University of Illinois Press.

Linden, D. J. (2011). *The compass of pleasure.* New York, NY: Viking Penguin Group.

McCann, L., & Pearlman, L. A. (1990). Vicarious traumatization: A framework for understanding the psychological effects of working with victims. *Journal of Traumatic Stress, 3*(1), 131–149. doi:10.1002/jts.2490030110

Miller, W., & Rollnick, S. (2002). *Motivational interviewing: Preparing people for change* (2nd ed.). New York, NY: Guilford Press.

Prescott, D. S., & Levenson, J. S. (2010). Sex offender treatment is not punishment. *Journal of Sexual Aggression, 16*(3), 275–285. doi:10.1080/13552600.2010.483819

Ray, M. A. (2010). *Transcultural caring dynamics in nursing and health care.* Philadelphia, PA: F.A. Davis.

Risdon, S., Wells, T., & Wesley, J. (2003). Opening the manager's door: State probation officers' stress and perception of participation in workplace decision making. *Crime and Delinquency, 49*(4), 519–541.

Simmons, C., Cochran, J. K., & Blount, W. R. (1997). The effects of job-related stress and job satisfaction on probation officers' inclination to quit. *American Journal of Criminal Justice, 21*(2), 213–217. doi:10.1007/BF02887450

Ward, T. A., & Gannon, T. (2006). Rehabilitation, etiology, and self-regulation: The comprehensive good lives model of treatment of sex offenders. *Aggression and Violent Behavior, 11*(1), 77–94. doi:10.1016/j.avb.2005.06.001

Watson, J. (n.d.). Caritas processes. Retrieved from www.watsoncaringscience.org

Watson, J. (2005). Caring science: Belonging before being as ethical cosmology. *Nursing Science Quarterly, 18*(4), 304–305. doi:10.1177/0894318405280395

Watson, J. (2008). *Nursing: The philosophy and science of caring* (Rev. ed.). Boulder, CO: University Press of Colorado.

Wong, P. T. (2011). Positive psychology 2.0: Towards a balanced interactive model of the good life. *Canadian Psychology/Psycholgie Canadienne, 52*(2), 69–81.

Zukav, G. (2014). *The seat of the soul* (25th ed.). New York, NY: Simon & Schuster.

# CHAPTER SIXTEEN

# Giving Voice Through Caritas Nursing

*Maryanne T. Sandberg*

## CARITAS QUOTE

*It is when nurses are able to authentically listen to another's story, to hold their suffering, for and with them, that may be the greatest healing gift. (Watson, 2012, p. 78)*

*This chapter describes how I used Caring Science in a special education classroom. Dr. Jean Watson's theory fit my instinctual identity as a nurse, validating the conviction that the nurse's caring presence is healing in itself. Concern about the deterioration of caring in nursing led me to become a nurse educator, striving to teach the art of compassionate care to my students. My work is based on the Caritas tenets of being authentically present, creative use of self, and allowing for miracles. I incorporated these tenets in my work with a medically fragile student who was unable to talk or write, severely limiting communication. Through the application of Watson's theory, I provided a healing environment that celebrated his life and enabled him to share his story. In turn, I learned important lessons about the art of nursing and living life to the fullest.*

## ■ OBJECTIVES

*The objectives of this chapter are to:*

- *Describe my personal discovery of Caring Science within my identity as a nurse*
- *Relate how Caring Science drew me to teaching*
- *Illustrate how I use Caring Science in my role as nurse/teacher*

## ■ JOURNEY TO CARING SCIENCE AND CARITAS LITERACY

My realization that Caring Science underpinned my practice came quite by accident. Caring Science has been part of my identity as a nurse and individual for as long as I can remember. Only I did not have a name for it until delving into nursing theory, where I found Watson's refined carative processes (Watson, 2008). Thirty years ago, as a young nursing student, I had studied Dr. Watson's theory with the original carative factors and recognized something familiar in them, but the meaning slipped away. My understanding was immature and the details of the theory escaped me, like a fleeting melody one cannot quite recall. I only knew that the essence of nursing was caring, and I wanted to project this to my patients. However, I was told to keep a protective wall between my patients and myself; that it was not professional to ever let my emotions show. Something inside my soul resisted. I knew I should not make my emotions the focus, but I also knew instinctively that there would be times when the most healing thing I could offer would be to share my patient's pain. I knew that if I wanted to connect with a patient, I needed to truly be there, my whole self, not just a professional shell.

Therefore, the concept of transpersonal caring relationships resonated strongly with me. I identified with the essence of connecting with patients on a far deeper level. Long ago I learned to enter patients' rooms mindful of how my presence was affecting them. Rushing in and out to do tasks does little to calm the spirit of the patient. I had learned that every patient in the hospital is scared, lonely, and in pain, whether physical or not. And most, at least at some level, are afraid they are going to die. It is a timeless moment when a nurse truly connects with a patient, sees the real self, listens deeply, and offers a caring presence to ease the pain, fear, and isolation that are often hidden below the surface. When I read, "It is when nurses are able to authentically listen to another's story, to hold their suffering, for and with them, that may be the greatest healing gift" (Watson, 2012, p. 78), it gave voice to the instinct I had been following. Dr. Watson's words validated my convictions about nursing. I had been practicing the art of transpersonal caring without knowing it, and there was deep satisfaction that I was not alone.

It was Caring Science that led me to become a nurse educator. My husband was hospitalized several years ago with pulmonary emboli. His experience in the hospital was not the best. Some of his nurses were compassionate, but there were several who were not. They treated my husband as if he was an object, rather than a real person in need of caring, not just physical care. The days he had those nurses were long, the 12 hour shifts stretching interminably. I was appalled by this lack of compassion. This reduction of care to duty-driven, technical treatments was not nursing, and I did not want my profession to continue in this direction. I believed I could help students to understand the art of nursing, not only the science; to know that truly being present with a patient does take time, effort, and intention, but it is an investment worth making. Nursing education then became my calling, and I have been teaching prelicensure students for 5 years. I emphasize what a responsibility and privilege we have as nurses to share in our patients' life-changing moments. I tap into the affective domain through the use of videos, but mostly I tell stories— stories about the patients who have made an impact in my life. I carry those moments of transpersonal caring with me as touchstones of nursing: treasures to share.

Caring Science also led me to one of my greatest adventures. I wanted to learn more about Watson's theory, so I looked for a conference that I could attend. There were no conferences in the United States for the time I was available, but there was a seminar in Lucca, Italy. Amazingly, I could go! It was a small, intimate gathering of extraordinary people, including Dr. Jean Watson. What a privilege to spend time with Caring Science Scholars and to hear their stories! We shared several days overflowing with love, beauty, healing, and joy in the golden Tuscan countryside. I was refreshed. I was energized. I was transformed.

## ■ KEY ELEMENTS OF CARING SCIENCE AND CARITAS RELATING TO TEACHING

I identify with many of the tenets of Caring Science, although there are a few in particular that guide my work. The first is being authentically present in my relationships with patients. The second is to use my full self as I care for them. And the last is to allow for miracles.

## TO BE AUTHENTICALLY PRESENT

Being authentically present means to offer an "intentional presence" that seeks to see the whole person, not merely the diagnosis or disease or even the physical body (Watson, 2012, p. 75). In other words, I am mindful that each patient (other) is a real person, with fears and problems, as well as talents and gifts. In caring for these patients, I am most effective if I can connect with patients on this deeper level. By recognizing and honoring who they are, greater healing can occur.

Being authentically present is not as mystical as it sounds. It means taking a moment to pause before entering the patient's presence to quiet oneself in preparation and focus on the nurse–patient relationship; to attend to all aspects of the patient, discovering what is meaningful to him or her; and to acknowledge these aspects by offering undivided attention to the patient's concerns, encouraging the patient to tell his or her story. Authentic presence also includes conversation about the patient's family or hobbies or even his or her favorite sports team. It is through these simple acts of respect and caring that we honor the patient for who he or she is as a person, not just a physical body. Authentic presence does not require any response from the patient. In fact, it is just as important, if not more so, to be authentically present with an unconscious patient or one who cannot communicate. I am convinced that the caring presence of the nurse has more healing power than we understand.

## TO USE ONE'S FULL SELF

Just as it is important to recognize the other as a whole person, it is important to acknowledge one's full self in the nurse–patient relationship. To use one's full self in caring for a patient means to respond to the patient as a full human being; as Watson (2012) asserted, "using every dimension of the person—all of one's unique gifts, talents, skills, knowledge, intuitions, tastes, perceptions, personality, and so on" (p. 77). In this way, I offer myself as part of the healing environment.

Once again, this is not as ethereal as it seems. I offer a cheerful, compassionate presence that is not forced, but rather comes from the heart. I can offer my humor as a means to help patients relax and let down their guard. And I can use my creativity to brighten the patient's environment, adding beauty and music to promote healing. Yet these are not the only means to offer one's full self. Each nurse brings unique talents that can be used to provide holistic care for patients. Often it is these moments of thinking and acting outside the box that result in the greatest healing of all.

## TO ALLOW FOR MIRACLES

The interaction of the whole patient and the whole nurse results in synergy. Thus, "this shared experience creates its own energetic phenomenal field and becomes part of a larger, deeper, complex pattern of life" (Watson, 2012, p. 79). Through caring interactions, both patient and nurse give and receive life-affirming energy, renewing each other's spirits. Sometimes these interactions result in even more: an inexplicable recovery, a moment of reconciliation, a precious chance to connect before a patient dies, or the comfort of a dream or vision.

Allowing for miracles does not mean to offer false hope. It simply means being open to possibilities beyond our imagining, to leave room for faith and hope, and to support these in our patients. These moments are difficult, if not impossible, to describe. It is more of a feeling than an event, when the nurse and patient transcend what is known and understood for a fleeting moment. Sometimes it can only be communicated through touch, or a glance, or the power of artistic expression. For me, the best way to communicate these miracles is through story.

## ■ HOW I IMPLEMENT CARING SCIENCE IN MY WORK

When I was invited to contribute to this book, my first thought was Nick. Before I started working as a nurse educator, Nick was a young man that I cared for as his long-term, one-on-one nurse so he could attend school. He was considered medically fragile, having been born with multiple deformities and health problems related to Holt–Oram syndrome, a rare genetic disorder. My duty was to monitor his health, provide physical care, and assist him with his studies. At age 17, he was just entering high school. We would be in a special education classroom. When I was offered the position, I was a substitute school nurse hoping for a permanent placement in one of the local schools. Working one-on-one was not what I had in mind, yet somehow I knew this was the job God had for me, so I accepted. I was concerned I would become bored caring for the same patient day after day. That was before I met Nick.

## EYES OF THE SOUL

I will never forget meeting Nick for the first time. Even after years as a nurse, his appearance took me by surprise. He was small for 17, and looked like a 10-year-old sitting in his large electric wheelchair. His body was contorted by severe scoliosis. He had a partial arm with a small hand and nubs for fingers on his right. On his left, he had only a partial hand with a few functioning fingers. His thin legs were obviously non–weight bearing and his feet rested on a footplate with several colorful buttons and a joystick. The wheelchair itself was bright orange. He had a feeding bag hanging on a pole attached to his wheelchair, because he could not eat. I knew he could not talk, and I could see that he rarely closed his mouth due to a large overbite. I took all this in at a glance, and then I saw his eyes. They were the most expressive eyes I have ever seen, filled with intelligence, apprehension, and hope. I knew at that moment I had made the right choice. I thought I was there to help Nick, to care for him and teach him. What I did not realize—what was impossible to fathom at that point—was how much he would teach me.

So Nick and I began our journey together. My first challenge was to learn to communicate with him. Nick had no problem understanding me. His ears worked perfectly. I, however, had some challenges understanding him. Several of the buttons on his footplate were connected to a voice box, which was tucked into a side pocket of his chair. He could move one leg and would press the buttons with his toe to say "yes" or "no." He could also turn his head to the left, indicating "yes," and to the right to say "no," and often used both his head and the buttons to emphasize his answer. Two other buttons had phrases recorded by one of his teachers. He could say, "My name's Nick" and "Hi, how are you?" He could also type, if his wheelchair was plugged into a computer. He would use the joystick as a mouse, selecting individual letters from an onscreen keyboard and clicking one of the buttons on his footplate. Typing was a laborious process, but he reveled in it. It was the only way he could express himself in words independently. His other means of communication was to gently nudge my leg with his toe to get my attention, signaling with his eyes that he wanted something. Usually, it was to go somewhere or to tell me something exciting had just happened. Behind thick glasses, his eyes looked enormous, his emotions plainly visible. Nick's eyes snapped with impatience to go on his visiting rounds in the school or shone with excitement about a pretty girl who was talking to him. I learned to read those incredible eyes and they were the basis of our communication. In essence, I learned that authentically listening to another's story does not always involve one's ears. Rather, it involves "intentional presence" (Watson, 2012, p. 75) and seeking with the eyes of the soul to see the spirit of the other.

## NICK'S VOICE

Another aspect of communication that was difficult for Nick was telling his family about his day at school. Nick's mother, Penny, would send a communication notebook into school every day. I used it to record when and how much formula Nick received, when he had bowel movements, any questions I had, or requests for supplies. Penny would reply, answering my questions or telling me about upcoming medical appointments or changes in Nick's routine. As I wrote in the notebook, Nick would often nudge me to tell me to write down about things he had done. Soon the notebook naturally evolved into a journal of his day, with Nick telling me what to include. He relished the ability to share with his family what he did each day. It became our routine for me to read the entry to him before he got on the bus so he could approve it. Penny treasured the notebook as well, and kept every page. When Nick got home each day, the first thing he wanted to do was to show his family the notebook. What had started out as a clinical nurse's notes and a necessary exchange of information was transformed into a window into his world: a glimpse of his life at school. He could finally answer the universal question, "How was your day?"

Nick had a mischievous sense of humor, so we began to experiment with his voice box to have some fun. Sometimes we would ask other people to record phrases for Nick. Although Nick was a Georgia boy, one day he would sound like a girl and the next he would have a Brooklyn accent. Nick found surprising others with his changing voices endlessly funny. We also recorded some of his favorite songs, so he could play music and dance, twirling his wheelchair around in time to the beat. During December we would record Christmas music, which I had to remind him not to play during class.

One day, one of his favorite teachers suggested he add a "Go Grizzlies!" to his recorded phrases to support the high school football team. Nick was excited by that idea and insisted that Mr. Martin record it for him. Mr. Martin was a gentle giant with a rich, deep voice, and was delighted to comply. From then on,

Nick and I would visit Mr. Martin weekly to have him record new phrases for Nick's voice box. Nick enjoyed startling people with a resounding, "No, no, no!" in his new booming voice. The two of them would conspire together to come up with ideas. Knowing Nick liked the girls, Mr. Martin would sometimes record lines like, "Hey, hey good looking!" or "Hi, there!" To Nick's total delight, he now had the words to go with his expressive eyes, and he used both to flirt shamelessly. As for Mr. Martin, he was honored to be the "Voice of Nick." Although we had a good bit of fun giving Nick new things to say, the voice box represented more than just funny phrases. It became a tool with which we could support the expression of Nick's feelings, helping to hold his story in words so he could share it more fully (Watson, 2012).

## CELEBRATING DIFFERENCES

One of the things I understood about Nick was that he wanted to fit in, just like any other teenager. Although he could not eat, we timed his feedings so that he could have his formula via his feeding tube at lunchtime, so he was "eating" with his friends. Sometimes I would put 60 mL of sports drink in his feeding bag to keep his electrolytes in balance. The addition of the sports drink would change the color of his liquid nutrition, which we jokingly referred to as a strawberry milkshake. He loved cruising around the lunch tables showing off his special drink. After all, no one else got milkshakes. It was the special education equivalent of being a "cool kid."

Another aspect of Nick's life that made him different from his friends was that he was incontinent and wore pull-on diapers. Although the students in Nick's classroom had cognitive impairment, they recognized differences just like other teenagers, leading to embarrassing questions about Nick's toileting habits. Emotionally, Nick was about 10 years old, but he was not mentally challenged, and he understood that although he was the oldest in the classroom, he was the only one wearing diapers. Occasionally, someone would make a comment like, "only babies wear diapers," and I could see the suffering and shame in his face. The teachers immediately addressed any unkind remarks, and had the offending student apologize to Nick, yet the pain still lingered in his eyes.

One day, after such an incident, I took Nick into the large closet that we used as a changing room. It was approximately 5 ft. by 10 ft. with windowless, cinder block walls. There was a changing table and a stack of drawers where we stored his supplies. It was blank and impersonal, almost like a prison cell. As I changed him, I talked to him about how many adults have to wear "pull-ups" just like him, and that wearing pull-ups did not mean that he was a baby. He turned his head left in agreement, but still looked miserable. As I held his suffering in my heart, I suddenly understood what to do, what needed to happen to create a healing environment for this young man.

"This room reminds me of my dorm in college," I said. "How would you like to make this your dorm room? You're the only student old enough to have one. We could decorate it, put up pictures on the wall, posters—whatever you want. What do you think?"

Nick's eyes shone with excitement. He strained his neck as far as he could to the left, which was his most excited "YES!" It was what Watson calls a caring moment, when the I-Thou connection between the nurse and other transcends understanding, creating a space for growth and healing (Watson, 2012). From then on, we collected things to decorate his dorm room. Bringing my camera to school, I took pictures of Nick and his friends and he chose ones to hang on the wall. Being a ladies man, his favorites were the ones of his "girlfriends." Nick also loved NASCAR, especially Tony Stewart. So together we chose pictures of Tony from the Internet to print and add to Nick's display. Word spread through the school about Nick's dorm room. Teachers, staff, and students brought him pictures, posters, and mementos to add to his wall. Together we created a sanctuary, with Nick guiding me wordlessly. No longer a room of shame, Nick's dorm room became an expression of his personality that he loved to show off to anyone and everyone.

## CREATIVE CARING

The high school Nick attended celebrated Halloween to the fullest. Teachers, staff, and students dressed up and competed for prizes. Creative energy permeated the school. It was not unusual to see groups of students dressed in coordinating costumes, such as parts of a Monopoly game. Of course, Nick wanted to join in the fun, so I would brainstorm ideas and he would say "yes" or "no." One year, his asthma flared as Halloween approached. He insisted on returning to school the day before the holiday, but Penny had not had time to find a costume. So he decided to be the same thing as the previous year: a chick magnet.

The year before Nick wore regular clothes with pictures of chicks taped all over him and everyone enjoyed the joke. It was fun the first time, but he was clearly disappointed with using the idea again. Repeating the same costume lost some of the luster. To make matters worse, he was still sick, wheezing and coughing. After a nebulizer treatment, we went on our visiting rounds. One of the secretaries at the main office said she had ordered a pirate costume for her grandchild and the company had sent two by mistake. She asked Nick if he would like to be a pirate and use the extra costume. Nick's eyes came alive with excitement. To his delight, the costume was Captain Jack Sparrow from *Pirates of the Caribbean*. As we returned to the classroom to show his teacher, I was inspired to take it to the next level. That night I went home and created a pirate ship out of a cardboard box that would cover his wheelchair. It had a figurehead, a cardboard ship's wheel, and, hanging from his feeding pole, sails and the Jolly Roger. The box completely covered his wheelchair with cutouts for the wheels, so that when he drove the chair he appeared to be sailing his ship.

Halloween was a big day, with Nick cruising the halls aboard his own version of *The Black Pearl*. He was so excited I could barely contain him long enough to give him his nebulizer treatments. At the end of the day, he took the costume home on the bus to show his family. Penny called me later, thrilled with his costume. She told me that Nick had driven all around their street showing off the pirate ship to the neighbors. I kept that message on my voicemail; it still makes me smile. It reminds me that sometimes the most therapeutic treatment is a cardboard pirate ship. Nebulizer treatments may have helped him breathe, but the pirate ship helped him live.

## SETTING THE SPIRIT FREE

I did give Nick quite a bit of nursing care during the 4 years I was with him. The nebulizer was a frequent companion, and despite his protests I had to send him home a few times when I could not manage his condition safely at school. We even rode together in an ambulance once when he became unresponsive. Yet as I look back on my nursing care, I realize that decorating his dorm room, playing with his voice box, and creating costumes were just as important for his health, if not more so. These simple acts contributed to the healing environment, potentiating Nick's wholeness as a person (Watson Caring Science Institute, 2010). Thus, Nick was able to express himself more fully, to join in the high school experience in all its camaraderie, raucous spirit, and youthful exuberance. Nick's vibrant personality was given a voice, and this set his spirit free. Even now, years later, I am humbled and honored to have had a part in this transformation.

## ■ REFLECTIVE PIECE

Nick died quietly in his sleep during the spring of senior year. He was 21 years old. He had long outlived his predicted life span, for which the doctors had no explanation. But I think Nick simply had things to do. He could not talk, or walk, or even eat, and spent most of his life in the same small southern town. Yet Nick affected more people, more deeply than most successful adults. Outside of his family, I think he affected me most of all.

Nick taught me that every person matters and has an important role to play in this life. In fact, sometimes the weakest of us all has the biggest impact. He taught me that life is a beautiful gift and it is meant to be celebrated. He taught me the true meaning of courage and friendship, to be thankful for the small things in life, to simply enjoy the ride. Nick also taught me how to be a better nurse. Acquiring the language and theoretical knowledge of Watson's Caring Science allowed me to reflect on my experiences with Nick and to understand them in light of the theory. I appreciate now what Dr. Watson means by the statement, "human-to-human caring relationships are mutual and life-giving and life-receiving for both nurses and others" (Watson, 2012, p. 11), because I received so much life from Nick. I understand the full use of oneself in caring for the patient, for there is so much more to nursing than physical care of the body. I learned there are many levels at which we can be authentically present with our patients and hear and support their stories, for it is through story that we come to be known and understand each other. And it is through holding another's story—both the joy and the suffering—that we honor each other and offer the greatest healing of all.

## ■ CONCLUSION

Nick continues to inspire and inform my caring practice and teaching. I remain open to the possibility of miracles, because I have seen them. Nick still brings miracles and joy into my life. Not too long ago I had a dream. I remember it vividly. I was walking in a sunlit field of swaying grasses. I saw a young man sitting on a large rock and stopped to talk to him. He was tall and strong and his eyes sparkled with mischief. Suddenly I recognized him, although he looked very different than the boy I cared for. "Are you Nick?" I asked, and he nodded, laughing. I woke up filled with joy.

Just recently I reconnected with Penny. I told her about my dream and she told me about others who had had similar dreams. Remaining open to the mysteries of life, we decided it must have been real. We talked about plans to write about Nick's life together, to continue to share his story. I look forward to the possibilities. I think we will enjoy the ride.

## ■ REFERENCES

Watson, J. (2008). *Nursing: The philosophy and science of caring.* Boulder, CO: University Press of Colorado.

Watson, J. (2012). *Human caring science: A theory of nursing.* Sudbury, MA: Jones & Bartlett.

Watson Caring Science Institute. (2010). Core concepts of Jean Watson's theory of Human Caring/ Caring Science. Retrieved from http://watsoncaringscience.org/files/Cohort%206/watsons-theory -of-human-caring-core-concepts-and-evolution-to-caritas-processes-handout.pdf

# PART SIX

# *Caritas Peace and Healing Arts*

In this inspiring section, nurses describe their work for peace, healing, and change in what could be called Emancipatory Caritas. Julie Benbenishty and Jordan Hannink describe the role of nurses as peacemakers in the Middle East by mediating conflict on the personal and societal levels. They describe a nonprofit organization called Nurses in the Middle East. This project originated from a small group of Israeli and Palestinian nurses who met with Dr. Watson and Ronald Lesinski of Watson Caring Science Institute in 2012 at the Peres Peace House in Jaffe, Israel. From that beginning emerged Middle Eastern Nurses Uniting in Human Caring, sponsored in part by Dr. Watson of the Watson Caring Science Institute and Israeli and Palestinian nurses. Beginning in 2013, four consecutive conferences, sponsored by Watson Caring Science Institute and HealingHealth with Dr. Susan Mazer and Dallas Smith, have been held in Jordan, allowing safe passage for Israeli and Palestinian nurses to come together. These conferences are now global, uniting nurses and others in human caring and peace throughout the Middle East and now from around the world. These conferences and this beginning organization have created safe space for leaders such as Mr. Suliman Turk, president of the Palestinian Nursing Council, and representatives from the Palestinian Ministry of Health to meet for shared problem solving and solution seeking toward common dilemmas threatening human caring for staff, patients, and citizens alike. These conferences provide the only opportunity for Palestinian nurses to have access to professional development outside the Palestinian territory and to communicate with each other. The new nonprofit Nurses in the Middle East helps to assure this shared work continues to unite nurses and others toward common goals of human caring and peace for the region. For more information on this unique program on caring and peace, see www.watsoncaringscience.org under Middle Eastern Nurses and Partners Uniting in Human Caring.

The chapter by Drs. Tsutsui, Emoto, and Watson informs readers of the remarkable 30-year history of Caring Science in Japan, including formal Caring Science curricula, pedagogies, research, creative scholarly projects, conferences, and research. Japan was one of the first countries in the world to be designated a Watson Caring Science Global Associate, Japan International Society of Caring and Peace, with participation in the co-creation of Watson Caring Science— World Portal Program Development.

In the final section, Dr. Mary Rockwood Lane describes her personal and professional experiences with Caritas healing arts, which led to the development of the first-of-its-kind Arts in Medicine program, involving 250 artists–poets– writers–dancers and others at a hospital in Florida, United States. This unique and inspiring program opened space for new expressions of human caring and the artistry of humanity. This original program paved the way for envisioning art as an advanced caring–healing modality for nursing interventions.

# CHAPTER SEVENTEEN

# Caring Practices in an Era of Conflict: Middle East Nurses

Julie Benbenishty and Jordan R. Hannink

## CARITAS QUOTE

*. . . [W]hen we proceed with knowledge and practices that others do not see, we then have a responsibility to offer it to others, to interrupt the world's pattern of violence and noncaring . . . there is a connection between Caring (as connecting with, sustaining, and deepening our shared humanity) and Peace in the world. (Watson, 2008, p. 49)*

*While the experience of conflict is not universal, we offer this chapter as a framework for looking at the ways in which conflict invades the health care system. Our hope, in doing so, is that nurses globally can apply key concepts to their own unique political and social landscapes. In recognizing that conflict exists in different forms, we chose to focus on Israel and Palestine, in order to achieve the depth necessary in applying theories of "peace through health" (Arya & Santa Barbara, 2008). We draw particular attention to hospitals in multicultural areas that receive high levels of traffic from all sects of society and clinics that are relatively homogenous.*

## ■ OBJECTIVES

*The objectives of this chapter are to:*

• *Describe ways in which Middle East nurses serve as peacemakers*

• *Explore continuity of care in this context*

• *Extend kindness and humanity*

• *Promote actionable research and cultural safety*

In Israeli hospitals, political conflict often plays out between hospital staff and the patient/family population. Ethnic, religious, and citizenship diversity among health care professionals, patients, and their families reflects the region's population, creating the potential for the hospital to work as a bridge to peace or as a powder keg.

Nurses are peacebuilders at the cellular level of disease and injury, like armies. Nurses are in charge of organizing the chaos of disease and "battling" accordingly. In addition to medical intervention, the nurse must assess the patient's mental state, ensure proper nutrition and hydration, and work toward mobility. Yet, the disease army does not operate without external allies and battlefield conditions. The nurse must consider the patient's identity, position in the family, and position in society. After initial assessment, nurses have to direct patients and their families on what the "new normal" will be. This may include extended time in the hospital or necessary accessibility changes that will need to be made indefinitely. The nurse then coordinates with a multidisciplinary team to streamline the patient's care plan with consideration for elements of holistic health that biomedical systems may ignore.

Simultaneously, nurses' care is inherently part of political and social conflict. Nurses are both representatives of the health system and of their individual identities. In cases where conflict permeates society, such as in Israel and Palestine, identity becomes a central factor for health workers, patients, and families. Rather than personal identity being "separated" from profession, nurses are aware of their identity, the identity of others, and find ways to mitigate potential problems. In other words, while systems of conflict enter the hospital, nurses create an atmosphere of new norms and values that leads to multicultural coexistence within the hospital (Goffman, 1961).

## ■ CROSSING THE BORDER: ISSUES OF MULTICULTURAL CARE

AA is a 45-year-old truck driver living in Hebron, West Bank. While driving a truck in Israel, he was involved in a head-on collision with another truck. He arrived at an Israeli hospital with life-threatening injuries.

During AA's hospitalization, Israeli authorities issued passes for his family to visit between West Bank and Israel, and his youngest brother was by AA's bed constantly. This brother only spoke Arabic and a little English, which limited communication between him and the health care team; however, he was included in discussions regarding AA's care.

After 3 weeks in an intensive care unit (ICU), AA recovered for another 2 months in the surgical department. During this time, AA was asked what he remembered about the accident and his ICU care. An Arabic-speaking nurse translated:

> I don't remember the accident at all. I do remember my dreams and nightmares during the time I was in ICU. I dreamt I was finally going to Haj Pilgrimage to Mecca (Pilgrimage—A journey made for spiritual reasons, often to a place of special religious significance). I spent months planning my trip delving into every intricate detail. I was very excited; a life dream was coming true. The week preceding my departure I spent hours with my wife planning the farewell dinner, we would sacrifice a lamb, grill the meat; there would be the best salads with the freshest vegetables, spicy rice, stuffed vegetables, and the most extensive honey coated baklava desserts filled with varieties of nuts. It is very traditionally significant that we have this family gathering. In ancient times those who set out for the Hajj had many hardships to overcome in order to travel to Mecca, and many did not return. This was a true farewell dinner. Friends close and distant relatives were all notified weeks before. We spent the entire day setting the table and arranging space for everyone to sit. We waited impatiently for our guests to arrive. No one came. I will certainly die on my Haj. (AA)

AA reported this delirious dream signifying many cultural aspects of this particular patient. His unconscious was plagued by worries that he would die in the ICU.

In addition, one can understand from this dream that AA felt socially isolated during his time in the ICU, which was triggered by the physical distance of his mother, wife, children, and extended family members. The importance of family in the Arab context intensifies the need of the family's presence for patient well-being.

After 3 months of total hospital length of stay, AA was ready to be released. His postdischarge treatment included care of his amputated stump, stoma care, remobilization, physical therapy, occupational training, and community reintegration, among other issues associated with posttraumatic return to life outside the hospital. Ideally, these ongoing medical concerns would be treated by therapists, nurses, and doctors in the community. These health care workers would have a full report on AA's case, understand the needed care, and be able to ask questions during a nurse-to-nurse handover.

This is not the case, however, in Israel/Palestine. Whenever patients have to be transferred for continued care in the Palestinian Authority or Gaza Strip, medical teams do not have the luxury of communicating with the next care team. AA's treating nurse, JB, did not know where to turn: She spoke with her Arab colleagues who worked in Israel but lived in the West Bank to attempt to establish contact with AA's next care team. She tried contacting nurses at a large hospital in the West Bank, and the Ministry of Health liaison; none of these efforts were successful. Unsatisfied with sending AA back into the world without ensuring continuity of care, JB attempted to maintain contact with the patient's brother and transmit medical information by phone through a translator.

The preceding case highlights several of the issues that arise as hospitals serve transnational patients. Differences in language, culture, and conflict experience require careful navigation by individual nurses and the nursing team. This example exemplifies challenges in caring practices in areas of political conflict.

## ■ CROSSING THE BORDER: LANGUAGE

While only context can affirm these numbers, communication psychologists often rely on the 55/38/7 formula, stating 55% of communication is body language, 38% is tone of voice, and 7% is the actual words spoken (Mehrabian & Wiener, 1967; Newcomb & Ashkenasy, 2002). Nonverbal communication is essential in creating the nurse–patient relationship, rooted in the establishment of trust. Nonverbal communication can either be intentional or unintentional. While intentional nonverbal communication conveys conscious thought, unintentional nonverbal communication often reveals subconscious thought. Unintentional nonverbal communication, such as hands on the hips, failure to make eye contact, or looking at your watch, can imply absence from the patient, which is detrimental to trust-building (Benbenishty & Hannink, 2015). In a recent study at a Jerusalem hospital, a Jewish nurse stated:

> "Because I don't think that language is a barrier—the barrier is if you are blinded by your own fears. And when you discover that the person in front of you is the same human being as you—the same needs, the same hopes, so this is how I think we could—and should—begin to live together." This example reflects the caring creative practice nurse[s] use to overcome and prevent conflicts when there are language barriers. (Jewish nurse, in Benbenishty & Hannink, 2015)

## ■ CROSSING THE BORDER: RELIGION AND TRADITION

There is a professional requirement for nurses to achieve competence in the delivery of spiritual care and to assess and meet the spiritual needs of their patients. Recently, the area of spirituality has come under criticism, bringing into question the role of the nurse with regard to the provision of spiritual care. If one traces the antecedents of nursing and health care, it is evident that these had a strong religious (Bradshaw, 1994) and spiritual heritage (McSherry & Jamieson, 2011).

Koenig and Larsen (2001) describe that it was religious communities that cared for the sick, destitute, and dying in a holistic integrated way. The findings imply that nurses, with or without a religious belief, consider providing competent spiritual care to be an integral part of their role. There seems to be an acceptance that, irrespective of one's own personal belief, there is a fundamental need to support patients to meet their spiritual needs (McSherry & Jamieson, 2011).

In our qualitative study of a Jerusalem hospital, an Arab nurse asserted:

> For example, I came to a patient to give him medication, and he said, "for the moment, I want to pray." So I said, "Okay, when you finish, tell me." I understand the importance of praying, so yes I pay attention to give respect to every culture and to respect religion in the hospital. But, in my opinion also, if it is an emergency, I will not wait until he prays. I explain to him, I will tell him that it is an emergency and I have to take care of him and after he can pray. Somebody who is calm, stable[,] I can tell him okay, you can pray, and after I can take care of you. It's a prioritization of what he needs, but it's important to me to give respect to all culture and all religion. (Arab nurse, in Benbenishty & Hannink, 2015)

Respecting religious practices is another manner in which nurses mitigate the potential clashes that may arise in the health care setting.

## ■ EAST MEETS WEST: UNDERSTANDINGS OF "HEALTH"

Conflicts are likely to occur whenever patients' health practices and beliefs differ from conventional Western care. For example, in the wave of Ethiopian immigration to Israel, Ethiopians held different beliefs on how the body functions. Similar to beliefs in the Evil Eye and other spiritual elements that create physical ailment, Ethiopian Jews hold different understandings of how disease enters the body (Hodes, 1997). In the case of a woman with hepatitis C, the nurse told her that her blood test reflected that her liver was diseased and required treatment. The patient asked, "What does my blood have to do with my liver?" While the initial reaction of medical professionals may be to explain their understanding of the body, it is more important to have the patient tell nurses and doctors how he or she understands his or her body. In doing so, disease, treatment, and healing options can be explained within the context that the patient understands.

Health education is dependent on cultural belongings. As we continue to globalize, Western medicine is either blended with or in opposition to traditional understandings of health and the body.

As the ideal marriage type in Arab Muslim society is between paternal first cousins (25%) and 75% of Palestinians marry some family relation, this results in an abnormally high rate of autosomal recessive disorders. One of these is Krabbe disease, which destroys the protective coating of the nerve cells in the brain and throughout the entire nervous system (Mayo Clinic, n.d.). The young infant is relatively normal, but around 6 months of age, feeding difficulties, unexplained crying, fever without infection, decline in alertness, delay in typical development milestones, muscle spasms, loss of head control, and frequent vomiting develop. The disease quickly progresses to include seizures, loss of development abilities, progressive loss of hearing and sight, rigid/constricted muscles, fixed posture, and progressive loss of the ability to swallow and breathe. Krabbe is incurable and treatment focuses on symptom relief. Most babies with Krabbe die before age 2, typically due to respiratory failure or complications from immobility.

The experience of having a sick child is draining on the mother in Arab society, where women are considered the caregivers. The frequent hospital stays, medication, additional health needs, and demand for constant care place a heavy financial and emotional burden on families. In addition to caring for a progressively disabled child, women are often blamed for their child's disease, as the disease is seen as passing from mother to child while in utero. In one case, a mother gave birth to three children with Krabbe, all of whom died before the age of 2. The woman's husband took a second wife, as his first wife's womb was cursed by the Evil Eye placed on the woman by jealous neighbors. In other cases, women were divorced after singular or multiple Krabbe births, because the women were seen as having "bad wombs."

Health care interventions in such cases require a refined cultural competency in order to provide the best care for each patient within the confines of tradition. Ultimately, a community nurse in one of the Israeli/Palestinian villages with a high rate of Krabbe worked with local clinics, nurses, imams, and higher Islamic authorities to advocate for abortion for babies diagnosed with Krabbe (earlier than 10 weeks). In more preventative measures, the local imam refused to marry anyone who had not been genetically tested or had high genetic probabilities of producing a Krabbe baby. Since this intervention 6 years ago, there has not been a single, new Krabbe case in this village.

In the same way that culturally competent care can relieve medical and social ills, poor cultural competency reproduces stereotypes and may lead to further microlevel conflict. The aim of cultural safety is to create an environment in which members of different groups feel safe to express and discuss their identity (Richardson & Carryer, 2005; Spence, 2005). However, the very act of raising issues that are connected with cultural safety can cause members of all groups to feel unsafe.

A study conducted on a mixed group of Arab and Israeli nursing students was a formative evaluation, using action research, of an academic nursing program in Israel. Part of this research was related to the integration of cultural safety education into the curriculum. The findings of the study showed that making it safe for minorities to present their culture to the majority group, dealing with the tendency of groups to deny the existence of conflict, making dynamics of oppression discussable, and creating conditions in which people can freely choose their individual and group identities were central challenges to be addressed in cultural safety education. The findings indicate that cultural safety education may engender painful issues that may make people feel unsafe. This does not imply that cultural safety education is not an important goal. On the contrary, the challenges that are described in this paper show how meaningful ethnic, national, and political identifications are for nursing students. It therefore indicates the importance of implementing cultural safety education in the nursing curriculum (Arieli, Friedman, & Hirschfeld, 2012). Understanding others and respecting traditional beliefs is yet another mode in which nurses mitigate conflicts before they erupt.

## ■ EDUCATED AS ENEMIES: OVERCOMING STEREOTYPES

Conflict in the Middle East is complex and requires more diligent research to fully understand its context than what can be offered here. Despite being political enemies, the Syrian Civil War and its proximity to Israeli hospitals compelled the State of Israel to accept those wounded by war into the care of Israeli doctors and nurses. Having Syrian patients was complicated by language, but more so by the two countries having a history of political animosity, raging wars, and constant hostility between them. Syrian patients, unlike Palestinians, had not had any contact with Israelis outside of stereotypes and media portrayals. Similarly, Israeli health care professionals were unaccustomed to treating Syrian patients.

In an Israeli hospital close to Syria's border, a nurse made this observation:

> Years of bloody civil war has caused thousands of Syrians to flee from their homes, and a few people caught up in the conflict and suffering found themselves in my country. Israel has considerable experience in dealing with the casualties of war and providing medical care for enemy soldiers. Syrian civilian casualties, however, are a new experience for the Israeli health service. One of our Syrian patients, Muchamed[,] is already acquainted with the staff of the internal medicine department. He has learnt all our names. His questioning eyes search our faces but we have no answers. We feel his anxiety. The complexity of life in the Middle East has brought us together. While the distances are small, we have grown up worlds apart. Now his loneliness and the tragedy of his diagnosis have connected us. The connection is a sincere one. We care about him, and we want him to mend and heal. Nursing and caring for the sick and wounded extends far beyond borders. In Israel, medical and nursing teams are ready and waiting at a second's notice to absorb and treat the wounded from Syria. We are willing and prepared to do what we can to meet their needs and ease their suffering. Our relationship, perhaps improbable, is, after all, a human one. Humanity seeks to restore peace where there is anxiety, kindness where there is cruelty and boundless love and care, where there is desolation and despair. Nurses are the true ambassadors of peace. (Israeli nurse, in Eisenberg & Benbenishty, 2013)

Frequent interaction between Syrian patients and Israeli Jews created trusting bonds, despite what politics, nationality, and religion dictated. Through trust building, the patient and the nurse were able to see each other as human beings in need of the same resources to maintain a good quality of life. Rather than being enemies, both leave the hospital with a greater understanding of that which is similar being more important than that which is different. Overcoming decades of enemy camps illustrates another aspect on a national/international level in which nurses demonstrate, in their role modeling, caring practices to calm conflicting stereotyping.

## ■ PRACTICAL APPLICATIONS OF CARING PRACTICES

Nurses, by making order out of the chaos of disease, have acted as conflict mitigators since the beginning of the profession. Practical applications for mitigating conflict through nursing are comprised in two parts—the first clinical, the second toward social justice. While both are patient-centered, they can also serve as models for interhealth care conflict.

In clinical settings, the nurse's presence sets the tone for relationship building or interpersonal conflict. When this coincides with caring across identity marker boundaries, it can either open conversations, expose vulnerability, and lead to trust, or it can reinforce stereotypes, which are detrimental to the nurse–patient relationship, patient healing, and relationships with greater society. Cognizance of presence on behalf of nurses includes reflecting on body language, tone, and acting with cultural competency. While we cannot assert nurses are not allowed "off days," we advocate for nurses reflecting on how their physical and emotional presence may affect others.

Structurally, health care settings can facilitate nurses' dual role as conflict mitigator by caring for nurses, providing burnout prevention, providing self-care rooms and staff support, and offering frequent debriefing with the aid of holistic healers, chaplains, and social workers. In the United States, some hospital staff members refer to the self-care process described as a "Code Lavender," which is used whenever a nurse has experienced a resuscitation or death during her shift. Rather than expecting nurses to continue healing other patients while pushing their own emotional wounds aside, a Code Lavender creates the space to recognize human emotions implicit in healing work. Hospitals could also offer resources for continuing education concerning cultural competency. Departmental nurses, for example, who specialize in cultural competency could be available for consultation, where medicine meets culture. Experts should be consulted on hospital decisions that have implications for diversity and on call to mediate conflicts between nurses and patients or between the hospital staff. Maintaining cultural competency teams allows nurses to apply their conflict mitigation skills without involving representatives from different strata of the health care hierarchy. Other interventions are nurse leadership training, focusing on team building in multicultural staffs, and arranging staff recreation and outings.

In our research, we found that the head nurse and nurse administrators are instrumental in creating space for multicultural staffs to flourish. Conversely, nurse leadership can isolate or cluster nurses based on identity, which results in distrusting relationships between nurses. By continuing to train nurses in leadership positions about multicultural team building, hospitals themselves demonstrate the possibilities for coexistence and partnership in larger society.

Nurses are also political actors outside of the hospital, with the potential to influence policy and social norms. As role models, nurses are obligated to have a code of behavior conducive to their profession. Some go beyond this call to try challenging systems that produce negative health outcomes, which include war, violence, abuse, and injustice (Arya & Santa Barbara, 2008). In the spirit of improving quality of life for all, a team of nurses from the Jerusalem area (including Hebron, Bethlehem, East Jerusalem, and West Jerusalem) has assembled with the goal of advancing patient outcomes across political and social borders. Nurses in the Middle East, a nonprofit organization, operates on the tenet that mutual caring has the potential to mediate the ways political oppression determines life chances and health outcomes. By working together on projects such as genetic disorder testing, early childhood injury, and alleged mistreatment of prisoners and terrorists in hospital settings, nurses involved have become not only colleagues but friends while bettering patient treatment and outcomes. As a young organization, they have already made an impact on the face of the Israel/Palestine health care world, and intend to continue. While recognizing their efforts may not solve the political conflicts, they maintain the potential for changing the ways the populations perceive each other. For the past 4 years, Dr. Jean Watson has supported the Middle East Nurses by providing financial support for nurses from low resource areas to attend the annual conferences. The mission statement of this nonprofit group is based on the Watson Caring Theory: Mission: "Middle Eastern Nurses Uniting in Human Caring promotes the practice and application of Caring Science/Caring theory for translating theory into concrete evidence-based approaches for self and others."

In this chapter, we have offered a new perspective for conflict mitigation. In our experiences as researchers, nurses often fail to recognize the magnitude their care has toward mediating conflict on personal and societal levels. Not recognizing such actions speaks to the ways that power and powerlessness have been reproduced in health hierarchies—since nurses are predominantly women and politicians predominantly men, nurses understand their potential for political impact through the lens of structural patriarchy. It is our intention that writing against this system of gendered oppression will encourage nurses to own their conflict mitigating powers from the cellular to global level. Second, we advocate for scholars to research nurses as essential to any political or social conflict resolution strategy. On an even larger scale, we aspire that soon nurses will not only have a place at the negotiation table, but also change the table altogether.

## ■ REFERENCES

Arieli, D., Friedman, V. J., & Hirschfeld, M. J. (2012). Challenges on the path to cultural safety in nursing education. *International Nursing Review, 59*, 187–193. doi:10.1111/j.1466-7657.2012.00982.x

Arya, N., & Santa Barbara, J. (2008). *Peace through health: How health professionals can work for a less violent world.* Bloomfield, CT: Kumarian Press.

Benbenishty, J. S., & Hannink, J. R. (2015). Non-verbal communication to restore patient–provider trust. *Intensive Care Medicine, 41*, 1359–1360.

Bradshaw, A. (1994). *Lighting the lamp: The spiritual dimension of nursing care. RCN Research Series.* Harrow, England: Scutari Press.

Eisenberg, S., & Benbenishty, J. (2013). Milk and rice. *International Nursing Review, 60*, 543–544. doi:10.1111/inr.12067doi

Goffman, E. (1961). *Asylums: Essays on the social situation of mental patients and other inmates.* New York, NY: Anchor Books/Doubleday.

Hodes, R. M. (1997). Cross-cultural medicine and diverse health beliefs: Ethiopians abroad. *Western Journal of Medicine, 166*, 29–36.

Koenig, H. G., & Larsen, D. B. (2001). Religion and mental health: Evidence for an association. *International Review of Psychiatry, 13*(2), 67–78. doi:10.1080/09540260124661

Mayo Clinic. (n.d.). Krabbe disease. Retrieved from http://www.mayoclinic.org/diseases-conditions/krabbe-disease/basics/definition/con-20029450

McSherry, W., & Jamieson, S. (2011). An online survey of nurses' perceptions of spirituality and spiritual care. *Journal of Clinical Nursing, 20*, 1757–1767. doi:10.1111/j.1365-2702.2010.03547.x

Mehrabian, A., & Wiener, M. (1967). Decoding of inconsistent communications. *Journal of Personality and Social Psychology, 6*, 109–114.

Newcomb, M., & Ashkenasy, N. (2002). The role of affect and affective congruence in perceptions of leaders: An experimental study. *Leadership Quarterly, 13*, 601–614. doi:10.1016/S1048-9843(02)00146-7

Richardson, F., & Carryer, J. (2005). Teaching cultural safety in a New Zealand nursing education program. *Journal of Nursing Education, 44*, 201–208.

Spence, D. G. (2005). Hermeneutic notions augment cultural safety education. *Journal of Nursing Education, 44*, 409–414.

Watson, J. (2008). *Nursing: The philosophy and science of caring* (Rev. ed.). Boulder, CO: University Press of Colorado.

# CHAPTER EIGHTEEN

# Japanese Caritas for Peace and Change[1]

Mayumi Tsutsui, Rina Emoto, and Jean Watson

## CARITAS QUOTE

*. . . a nurse or a nurse student must first treat self with gentleness and dignity prior to caring for patients, families and communities. . . . (Watson, 1985)*

*This chapter highlights some of the elements of Caritas Literacy in Japan that were introduced over 20 years ago. A backdrop of developments in Japanese Caring Science Theory, including programs and activities, is offered as an historic context, reflecting devoted Japanese scholarship in Caring Science Theory since the mid-1980s. Next, the chapter emphasizes the more recent caring and peace initiatives beginning with the First International Hiroshima Caring and Peace Conference, held in Hiroshima at the Red Cross Hiroshima College of Nursing, March 2012. The final section summarizes two Caring Theory–guided research studies that provide a pattern for Caritas Literacy in relation to the caring environment.*

---

[1] For more information on global activities in Japan and elsewhere, visit Jean Watson and the Watson Caring Science Institute (www.watsoncaringscience.org)—the site includes videos of the International Hiroshima Caring and Peace Conference.

## ■ OBJECTIVES

*The objectives of this chapter are to:*

• *Describe the historic background of major Japanese Caring Science initiatives, programs, and projects*

• *Increase understanding of personal/professional Caring Science developments in Japan*

• *Provide exemplars of Japanese initiatives and scholarship*

## ■ JAPANESE CARITAS FOR PEACE AND CHANGE

As early as 1989, Dr. Watson was invited to keynote the First Scientific Nursing Research Conference in Tokyo, Japan. This event, along with caring theory books being translated into Japanese and annual student/faculty visits to the University of Colorado to meet Dr. Watson and others from the mid-1980s, is reflective of early interest in caring theory and Watson's Caring Science. In December 2000, Dr. Watson was invited to once again present the keynote presentation to 3,000 Japanese scholars attending the 28th Academic Conference of the Japan Academy of Nursing Science under the leadership of Dr. Yasukata (yasukata@ndmc.ac.jp).

In 2012, immediately prior to and coordinated with the *International Hiroshima Conference on Caring and Peace*, the Japanese Red Cross College of Nursing (in Tokyo) hosted a formal presentation during which Dr. Watson was awarded an honorary doctorate. This occasion was a reflection of the more than 20-year history of Japanese Nursing and Red Cross Colleges' (in both Hiroshima and Tokyo) commitment to the development of knowledge, values, philosophies, theories, and practices of human caring. Dr. Fumiaki Inaoka; his wife, Mitsuko Inaoka; and Ms. Michiko Tomura were translators of the first Japanese edition of Watson's original theory book: *Nursing: Human Science and Human Care: A Theory of Nursing* (1985). Dr. Tsutsui translated Watson's *Assessing and Measuring Caring in Nursing and Health Sciences* (2001).

Adoption and implementation of Caring Science is ongoing in Japan. Examples include formal Caring Science curricula, pedagogies, research, creative scholarly projects, conferences, and research. Of note, a Center for Human Caring was created in the Hiroshima Red Cross College of Nursing as early as 2000. Watson's books—*Measuring Caring, Postmodern Nursing,* and the original and revised *Human Caring Science* texts—have been translated into Japanese since the mid-1980s, reflecting a 30-plus-year interest and collaboration in Caring Science. Dr. Watson was invited to present the inaugural keynote address at the establishment of the Japanese Red Cross Hiroshima College of Nursing in 2000.

Since the 2012 International Hiroshima Conference on Caring and Peace, a new International Collaborative Center has been created at the Japanese Red Cross College of Nursing (in Tokyo). It is led by Dr. Mayumi Tsutsui, who is a Caring Science Scholar and regular participant in Caring Science programs in the United States and throughout Japan. Dr. Watson returned at the request of Japanese nurses to deliver a second keynote address at the Second International Conference on Caring and Peace, November 2015. (The Third International Conference on Caring and Peace will be held on March 25–26, 2017.)

More recently, in 2016, a new *International Society of Caring and Peace* has been established, with Dr. S. Shindo as the new president/chair (Dr. Jean Watson, Honorary Chair Emerita) providing continuity from the 2012 Conference, where Dr. Shindo served as conference moderator and chair. These personal/professional connections and formal scholarly Caring Science occasions have continued since 1989 to the current moment.

The newest innovation extends the collaboration between Dr. Watson and Japanese nurses. Japan was one of the first countries in the world to be designated a Watson Caring Science Global Associate, Japan International Society of Caring and Peace, with participation in the co-creation of Watson Caring Science—World Portal Program Development (2016–2018, www.watsoncaringscience.org).

## ■ EXEMPLARS OF JAPANESE SCHOLARSHIP AND CARING SCIENCE LEADERSHIP

With this background of personal/professional history of Japanese Caring Science scholarly evolution, the next section emphasizes the caring and peace global conferences and continuing commitment to caring and peace.

## INTERNATIONAL HIROSHIMA CARING AND PEACE CONFERENCE— MARCH 2012

The early leaders for the 2012 Caring and Peace Conference include Dr. Shindo, president of the Japanese Red Cross Hiroshima College of Nursing at that time; Dr. Inaoka, former inaugural president of the Japanese Red Cross Hiroshima College of Nursing and moderator–host of the Watson Caring Science Institute, First Asian Pacific International Caritas Consortium prior to the Caring and Peace Conference; it is also imperative to acknowledge and name Ms. Michiko Tomura, devoted Caring Science faculty in the Japanese Red Cross Hiroshima College of Nursing, a major leader with all the evolution of Caring Science in Japan, and currently a doctoral student in the United States.

## SUMMARY OF 2012 CONFERENCE—ADVANCING CARITAS LITERACY IN RELATION TO PEACE

This 2012 International Hiroshima Conference on Caring and Peace brought forth new intellectual–experiential scholarly connections between human caring and peace. That is invoking a Caritas Literacy consciousness that practices of human caring are indeed practices of peace.

The ancient land of Japan and Hiroshima, the city of world peace as well as the site of the Hiroshima Peace Memorial Museum, provided a perfect setting for this first of its kind conference. Here, the conference opened by fire from the sacred mountain on the Island of Miyajima, radiating the light of caring and peace to all present and to all caring practitioners around the world.

The Caritas Literacy rhetorical questions, which arose from the opening conference keynote—*Touching the Heart of Our Humanity: The Caritas Path of Peace* (Watson, 2012)—were as follows:

- What is peace?
- What is the origin of peace?
- What is inner peace? How do we obtain it?
- How do we manifest and sustain human caring and peace in our heart, mind, and daily acts?
- Is there a connection between inner peace and outer peace?
- How do we offer up our hearts to caring and peace when there is so much pain in our hearts and in our world?

The approach to these rhetorical yet universal Caritas Literacy questions was addressed through philosophical–ethical and practical ideals from the Latin notion of Caritas and Caring Science (Watson, 2012):

> We as nurse and health professionals know, that when we step into the theories and philosophies of human caring, we step into a deep ethic and life practice that connects us with the heart of our humanity, of healing the whole; it is here in this connection, we touch the mystery of inner and outer peace that unites humanity across time and space around the world.

Indeed, this Japanese conference affirmed that Caritas Literacy, as addressed in this book, includes human dignity, basic civility, and humanity, which is peace in action.

This Hiroshima conference created Caritas Literacy experiences, space, and intellectual discourses whereby the audience engaged in awakening of Caritas consciousness—awakening to the reality that when we offer our own life, one person to another, finding more conscious intentional ways to live, gestures of peace within and without, then we become caring/we become peace/we are peace. We become a living beacon of hope and action for Caritas Literacy in relation to caring and peace for our world. Living and speaking Caritas Literacy generate peace from within. As such, this 2012 Japanese conference laid the global foundation for nurses to participate in co-creating a moral community of caring and peace for our world.

## JAPAN—CONTINUING CARITAS

The 2012 International Hiroshima Conference on Caring and Peace was a prelude to the more recent works in Japan including the new international society and projects. The Caring Science Institute has supported the creation of an ethical–scholarly professional community of caring scholars and practitioners. Likewise, Japan held its Second International Conference on Caring and Peace in the Fall of 2015, and the third one is already scheduled for March 2017.

A continuation of these global Caritas Japanese activities includes the 2016 creation of the International Society of Caring and Peace, formally extending Caritas into the Asia Pacific and beyond. Dr. Mayumi Tsutsui, coauthor of this chapter, is a founding member of the new International Society of Caring and Peace, allowing this momentum to live on.

In summary, these grassroots Japanese efforts continue to attract nurses and health professionals from around the world; together, they stand as beacons for global initiatives, reflecting the Caritas Literacy initiatives informing this book. For more information on both the Japan conferences go to www.watsoncaring science.org under Global Programs. In the next section, we provide two exemplars of Caritas scholarship in Japan.

## ■ CARITAS LITERACY RESEARCH EXEMPLARS

### JAPANESE RED CROSS COLLEGE OF NURSING—TOKYO RESEARCH PROGRAM: INTEGRATIVE REVIEW

Drs. Tsutsui and Emoto and their colleagues from the Japanese Red Cross College of Nursing conducted what may be considered first-generation Japanese research on Caring Science. This Caring Theory–guided Japanese research study was conducted in two phases. In the first phase, the authors conducted an integrative review focusing on literature relating to Watson's Caring Theory (Tsutsui, 2011).

CINAHL, Full Text, and ICHUSHI (Japan's medical databases) were searched from 2000 through July of 2010. The studies of human caring were examined carefully for fit with the intended purposes of this project. Thirty-two studies were relevant to the assessment made through methodological qualitative–quantitative inquiry of the caring environment. The findings identified four steps of creating an environment for caring and substantiated several aspects of Watson's theory:

- A nurse or nurse student must first treat self with gentleness and dignity prior to caring for patients, families, and communities
- Nurses benefit from participation in a Watson theory session, offering intensive, purposive support to translate theory into daily clinical nursing practice

- The caring theory intensive may be a contributing factor to a patient's perceptions of nurses and satisfaction with health care services
- Even though technology has advanced, caring is the value that inspires nursing and development of patient care with the team

In the second phase, the authors explored a synthesis of Watson Caring Science as a guide to creating–healing environments on pediatric wards in a medical setting and was approved by the Japanese Red Cross College of Nursing Ethics Committee. The focus of this inquiry was to assess what aspects of Watson's Theory of Human Caring create an environment for caring (Tsutsui, 2010).

## JAPANESE RED CROSS COLLEGE OF NURSING—TOKYO RESEARCH PROGRAM: CREATING A CARING ENVIRONMENTAL MODEL

The results of the integrative review yielded the previously mentioned four steps to creating a caring environment. Next, the researchers conducted a study using a participatory action research (PAR) intensive designed to help nurses explore the Caritas Processes and their effects on the nurse, the child, and the health care experience (Emoto, Tsutsui, & Kawana, 2015).

The background of this work is based on cultural norms. In Japan, even though people may have a need to ask questions, they may be hesitant to do so, because they are likely to believe that it can affect their relationships with others by being perceived as burdensome or overly assertive. Because harmonious interpersonal relationships are highly valued, direct confrontation is avoided whenever possible. There is a reliance on the sensitivity of the other person to pick up the point of the conversation.

The pediatric ward is very busy. As children's verbal and cognitive abilities are in the process of development, assessment of the child's condition is very difficult. Caring for children takes more time than for adults, accounting for time to explain and engage children in the various treatments. At the time of the PAR, Japanese nurses discussed patients and families in care conferences; however, there was no opportunity to discuss professional practice issues that impacted their confidence in caring for children. As a result, clinical and practice challenges remained "buried," sometimes negatively impacting nurses' satisfaction with their own performance and their jobs.

The researchers conducted PAR in six hospitals in Japan in six pediatric wards and one pediatric outpatient department. The study was approved by the Ethics Committee of the Japanese Red Cross College of Nursing. The researchers recruited six master's prepared clinical nurse specialists with greater than 5 years of experience as co-researchers. In turn, the co-researchers recruited nurse members; together, they designed the research collaboratively. The groups held discussions and data were used from the narrative discussions and other sources. The data were rich descriptions of nurses' clinical challenges. The discussions identified issues that nurses were facing silently due to cultural norms. For example, one pediatric nurse received harsh words from a pediatric patient and family. Although she wondered what she did to deserve being treated in such a way, she suppressed her feelings and continued to provide care. The nurse who was hurt by the patient's/family's harsh language had difficulty talking about the experience because she believed that telling about feeling hurt "would result in being labeled as being an incapable nurse," and "revealing my true feelings and saying something improper is not what a good nurse is supposed to do." She eventually began talking and revealed that she had tried to maintain a distance from the child and the family but that her work motivation diminished. The session resulted in peers sharing similar experiences and feelings. They empathized with her feelings without denying them and helped her regain the motivation for providing care. After 8 months, the healing experience of nurses resulted in improvements in care among children and families.

We need to care for ourselves, without being held back by fixed ideas like what a nurse *should be*. Participating in PAR provided ongoing opportunities in which nurses could talk about their feelings without hesitation. Nurses found these sessions invaluable. They felt cared for by their superiors and the organization. They felt more able to care for patients/families in ways that could facilitate health and healing.

The results of ongoing dialogue about challenging situations allowed nurses to share negative experiences that were undermining their confidence. To improve the situation, nurses were given mutual understanding between staff nurses. As a result of dialogue, nurses were released from negative experiences. Identity crises were changed to competencies and nurses expressed more passion for nursing. The model that was developed as a result of this research showed an iterative relationship between the Caritas Processes, healing nurses, redefining existing problems, and disclosing hidden problems.

This action research was supported by one of Dr. Watson's carative factors, "the provision for a supportive, protective, and (or) corrective mental, physical, sociocultural, and spiritual environment" (carative factor 9) and was found to be key to a secure and safe caring environment for the care provider. This study was supported by the Grant-in-Aid for Scientific Research from the Ministry of Education, Culture, Sports, Science, and Technology for the fiscal years of 2007 to 2010. Dr. Watson served as a research mentor in these studies.

## ■ CONCLUSION

This chapter has provided an historic overview of Japanese developments and interest in Caring Science and Theory of Human Caring over the past 30 years. For example, the first foreign translation of Watson's Theory of Human Caring was in Japanese (translated by Fumiaki Inaoka [Watson,1985]). Japanese nursing has been a leader in academic–research scholarship as well as projects and programs in Caring Science Theory. Another example is that the Japanese Red Cross Hiroshima

College of Nursing was inaugurated with Caring Science Theory as the basis of its curriculum and Dr. Watson was the inaugural keynote speaker. This was followed by the establishment of the Japanese Red Cross Hiroshima College of Nursing Center for Human Caring, which was modeled after the Center for Human Caring, University of Colorado, in the 1980s.

As the focus on Caring Science advanced in Japan, the first Japanese research conferences included a Caring Science Theory focus and featured Dr. Watson as a keynote speaker (1989). This culminated in the Japanese Red Cross College of Nursing (in Tokyo) awarding Dr. Watson an International Honorary Doctorate (2012), followed by the Japanese Red Cross Hiroshima College of Nursing sponsorship of the First Asian Pacific International Caritas Consortium and the First International Hiroshima Caring and Peace Conference.

These historic beginnings are continuing up to the current time, embracing the Second International Conference on Caring and Peace, Tokyo (2016), with dates scheduled for March 2017. Finally, the chapter closes with an overview of extant caring theory research, which provides some guidelines for Caritas Literacy—Japan, in relation to the caring environment. The PAR was an important milestone in Japan, helping nurses care for each other, thus creating a caring–healing environment for all.

## ■ REFERENCES

Emoto, R., Tsutsui, M., & Kawana, R. (2015). A model to create a caring and healing environment for nurses in child and family. *International Journal for Human Caring, 19*(1), 8–12.

Tsutsui, M. (2010). *Environment creation of caring and healing in pediatric nurses: Nursing action research* (Research Report of 2007–2010). Grant-in-Aid for Scientific Research, Ministry of Education, Culture, Sports, Science, and Technology, Tokyo, Japan.

Tsutsui, M. (2011). Caring in nursing: Its trends and perspectives. *Journal of Nursing Research, 44*(2), 115–128.

Watson, J. (1985). *Nursing: Human science and human care: A theory of nursing* (F. Inaoka and M. Inaoka, Japanese Trans.). Sudbury, MA: Jones & Bartlett.

Watson, J. (2001). *Assessing and measuring caring in nursing and health sciences* (M. Tsutsui, Japanese Trans.). New York, NY: Springer Publishing.

Watson, J. (2012). *Touching the heart of our humanity: The Caritas path of peace* [Keynote address]. International Hiroshima Conference on Caring and Peace, Hiroshima, Japan.

CHAPTER NINETEEN

# Caritas Arts for Healing

Mary Rockwood Lane

## CARITAS QUOTE

*Upon awakening each day, begin with spiritual practice, even if it is being silent to receive the day and to give gratitude for life. Be open to receive the day and all the universe wishes you to receive and give in return. Set your intentions. Bring your full self, your presence in the moment. Establish your intentions. Be guided by caring, compassion, tenderness, gentleness, loving kindness and equanimity for self and others. (Watson, 2002, p. 18)*

*For many years, my personal and professional lives have been guided by Caring Science. In this chapter, I describe my own healing through painting and how that experience informed the first-of-its-kind Arts in Medicine program, of which I was the cofounder and codirector. The program, which began from a bone marrow transplant unit at Shands Hospital, expanded to other units and became a national model for integrating the arts into health care. I am an associate faculty at the Watson Caring Science Institute and University of Florida School of Nursing, where I teach Creativity and Spirituality in Healthcare. To learn more, see www.maryrockwoodlane.com.*

## ■ OBJECTIVES

*The objectives of this chapter are to:*

• *Describe my journey to Caritas*

• *Demonstrate how once I experienced the healing power of art, I created the first-of-its-kind Arts in Medicine program that became a national model*

## ■ JOURNEY TO CARING SCIENCE AND CARITAS

I remember when the journey began. There was a moment of recognition, and simply no words. It was like seeing a shooting star fly across the vast spacious dark night-time sky. I saw her radiance. I was in awe. It was magical. An exquisite beauty that takes your breath away. In that moment I recognized something incredible and rare.

That moment evolved during a conference in Toronto, Ontario, Canada, in 1984. It was a large nursing theory conference in the heyday of theory in nursing academics. There were literally thousands of nurses in attendance. I was thrilled to be at the theory conference in Canada. Martha Rogers, Virginia Henderson, Rosemarie Parse, and many nursing giants were there. I was motivated and felt really excited about my whole future in the nursing profession. During the conference, I was just open and listening to the lectures.

I remember the moment I wandered into a large auditorium and looked up on the stage to see a woman surrounded in a soft, radiant light. The room was large, dark, and crowded. I stood in the back, and suddenly the soft light expanded into the room. The energy was peaceful. There was a deep sense of quiet, trust, and calm as she spoke. I listened to the primal sound of her voice as she spoke in the midst of chaos of a large conference that was filled with so many speakers and participants. I listened with my heart, not my mind. I remember how I felt—calm, centered, and quiet. I do not remember her words; I simply remember her presence. I stood still and watched; she was glowing and surrounded in soft translucent white light. The light was shining from her and around her form, about 3 to 4 ft. in a sphere of light. It was beautiful. Somehow it filled the whole room. It was like an invisible light that flowed from an energy field that expanded and reached across the entire space and touched everyone in the room. She stood up, bringing in the light. All I felt was love and light. I did not know who she was. I remember asking a woman standing near me who she was. She spoke her name but I did not remember; I had seen a light like that around a person before. It was beautiful. She was a holy and blessed human being. The light was vibrating at a higher frequency. I felt touched by her presence. It was so subtle, soft, and tender. The time slowed down. I took a deep breath. That was my first memory of her. Many, many years later, when I looked back, I realized that was the first time I ever saw Dr. Jean Watson.

## BEGINNINGS

I graduated from the University of Florida in 1977. As a new graduate nurse, I worked at Beth Israel Hospital in Boston. I loved nursing and discovered a great profession. When I returned to graduate school at Boston College, I discovered theory, research, and how much I loved learning. Nursing was a rich and evolving science.

There was a thrilling intellectual community in Boston. At that time in my life, I worked directly with Joan Borysenko, PhD, a leading authority on stress, spirituality, and the mind/body connection. Dr. Borysenko was then completing her third postdoctoral fellowship in psychoneuroimmunology with Dr. Herbert Benson, author of *The Relaxation Response* (Benson, 1975). In 1978, Bernie Siegel, MD, originated *Exceptional Cancer Patients*, a specific form of individual and group therapy utilizing patients' drawings, dreams, images, and feelings (Siegel, 2011). Jon Kabat-Zinn, PhD, founding executive director of the Center for Mindfulness in Medicine, Health Care, and Society, as well as the founding director of the Stress Reduction Clinic at the University of Massachusetts Medical School, was just beginning his work in stress management and meditation (University of Massachusetts Medical School, 2014). So, within that context and rich intellectual history, I conducted my master's thesis on the relaxation response, stress management, and making images with patients suffering from chronic pain. It was the cutting edge of a paradigm shift in pain and stress management. It was the most exciting place and time to be a new nurse.

## FALL INTO DESPAIR

I returned home and literally disappeared into my life. My husband and I left Boston when he finished his residency and we settled back to Gainesville, Florida, my home town. I found a job as an instructor at the University of Florida College of Nursing, where I taught for about a year and a half before delivering my second child. I decided to stay home to be a mother. It was the hardest thing I ever had done.

That job at home was my first failure; I was not happy. I was not cut out for the intensity of motherhood. My husband worked constantly as he was starting his new surgery practice. My children were 2 years apart and I needed help. We built a new home and I managed the best I could.

As a nurse, I had become someone. I was capable, confident, and highly motivated. I had met my husband when he finished medical school. I moved away to Boston. I got a fabulous job at the Beth Israel hospital in primary nursing. I worked on a step-down cardiac unit. I loved my patients. I loved being a nurse. My master's degree at Boston College prepared me to become a primary care clinical specialist, having expertise in alternative holistic therapies. I became a certified nurse practitioner in primary care. I worked as a health care provider in my own nursing practice in the out-patient gynecology clinic. I loved working, loved learning, and loved the beauty of a structured and consistent life pattern. I found my strength, my creativity, and my independence.

When I was home with two small children, my life changed. My life unraveled and I was struggling to keep my head above water. I entered a place of deep despair and profound depression. I wanted to be a good mother more than anything. But, I needed help for the first time in my life. And, I collapsed. I was not good enough to be a mother. I was ashamed, unequipped, and inadequate. This created shame and disappointment in myself, which I was not prepared for.

## PAINTING MY WAY TO WHOLENESS

Eventually, I went through a severe depression during a 2-year marital separation. I felt like I was drowning as the therapy was not helping. I always dreamed of being a painter but I did not feel I could ever be good enough. But, in the depths of my outrage and depression, I decided to abandon all of my fears of being a painter. My first painting was inspired by a photo in a magazine of a woman who was distorted; this began a series of self-portraits in which I painted my pain with purely emotional intensity. Later, when I saw the first self-portrait, I realized that the painting captured the genuine expression from a moment in time that was now *behind me*. As I immersed myself in painting, I realized that I was healing. "By seeing my pain on canvas, I could step away from it" (Rockwood Lane, 2010).

## IN DIVINE ORDER

My professional journey was born out of the power of that experience, that suffering, and the despair. After that period, my life transformed from the void of darkness to something larger than myself. Everything was in Divine order. I discovered my life's work out of a personal healing experience. This was how I discovered my calling and my life's purpose. The experience of becoming and being a Caritas nurse/person comes from this personal story and living the theory.

When I began my doctoral studies, I discovered Dr. Watson's work. During the first call I made to inquire about the doctoral program, I discussed my interests with Dr. Sally Hutchinson, who would become my dissertation chair. In our first conversation, I was telling her about my experience of art and healing, and that I wanted to expand nursing practice and do phenomenological research. Dr. Hutchinson listened and said, "First, go visit Jean Watson." So I did.

Caritas became the guide of my whole life and the work has cultivated my way of being and knowing. The theory became my very foundation and my philosophy in life, my spiritual practice, and the essence of my being. It was essential for me to *practice* to become caring with my whole being so I could evolve as a human being. It was a process to become healed, empowered, and to make a contribution to my profession. My intention was to become a better human being, and finally forgive myself for not being the mother I wanted to be. Caring Science became my religion, my understanding, my lens to see the world, and what I wanted to accomplish as part of my life destiny.

## ■ HEALING WITH THE ARTS

The overarching tenet of Caring Science that impacted my life and nursing practice was that caring happens in the energetic unitary field of consciousness and that field is love (Watson, 2012). My life's work had become Healing With the Arts. I had healed myself by creating art and painting a series of self-portraits. This powerful creative healing process led to my vision to create an Artist in Residence program at the local teaching hospital at the University of Florida. The universe was calling on my life to manifest this dream of integrating the arts into health care. I was inspired and guided by creativity, compassion, and love.

When I met Jean Watson in 1991, her work resonated deeply. I knew it as my reality and the Theory of Caring Science was the language to describe what I already knew to be true. Jean introduced me to Alex Grey's visionary art. I read all her books, and went to see Alex's work in New York City. I studied extensively. My destiny unfolded in a moment. I was connected to something larger. Jean Watson was the dean of the School of Nursing at the University of Colorado. All I needed was affirmation and I got it. I was ready to change the world. The theory was my grounding, my secret knowledge, my empowerment, my strength, and my understanding of how to move forward. Caring Science provided the moral, metaphysical, ontological, philosophical, and scientific worldview (Watson, 2008). It presented working assumptions to relocate my professional knowledge and myself in practice.

## LOVING-KINDNESS

The major element of the Theory of Human Caring that has impacted my life the most intensely has been the practice of loving-kindness (Watson, 2008). This would be my greatest challenge to transform my being. My commitment was to embody Caritas with my whole being: in my mind, emotions, body, and spirit. This has become my practice for personal and professional growth. This would become my deepest spiritual commitment that would require my whole life to practice every single day. This Caritas Process became my guidepost and my mantra. Centering and practicing with my singing bowls would become my daily touchstone. This is my spiritual practice; deepening my heart connection is my starting point to begin each day. I know what I hold in my heart is important. Jean's words and Caritas Processes (Watson, 2008) are my daily intentions. Dr. Watson is a real human being, a living mystic, and the Oracle returning. She is my teacher and a best friend.

# ■ CARING–HEALING ACCOMPLISHMENTS

## ARTS IN MEDICINE

My initial theory-guided project was creating the first-of-its-kind Arts in Medicine program in 1991. Described in the following text, this became a national model of arts integration into health care and was based in Caring Science.

Caring Science views the cosmos as sacred. Nursing practice would create the sacred space in the health care delivery system. It would be the umbrella of the clinical practice model. The inspiration to bring the arts back into the health care/healing process was a return to an ancient path; remembering another way of being. This was a dream larger than any one person; the time that had come. There were many people—artists, nurses, physicians, social workers, and hospital administrators—called to return and to create this re-patterning of the health care field. It was about the return to the Divine Feminine, in the midst of a hard scientific medical business masculine model of health delivery (Watson, 1999). This Caring Science, joined to the arts, was about a new mystic/spiritual worldview. The unitary field of consciousness was evolving, opening, and reorganizing for change to emerge.

The Arts in Medicine program began in the nursing department of a teaching hospital; a contemporary patient care initiative. For more than a decade, Caring Science guided my contribution as the codirector of the artist in residence program. My program evolved because caring was the essential foundation for health care; the art/artist events were embraced by the clinical nursing staff. The Arts in Medicine program demonstrated the power of caring. Caring was the underlying disciplinary, philosophical, theoretical base encompassing art as part of the clinical environment.

The Arts in Medicine project was co-led by John Graham Pole, MD. Our nurse/physician partnership extended to the hospital's chief operating officer, chief nursing officer, and the nursing director of the bone marrow transplant unit. As an interdisciplinary leadership team working with the nursing staff, we explored many possibilities such as introducing the art activities as advanced nursing therapeutics. We conducted unit-based workshops and sought nurses' feedback about how to integrate the art activities with families and patients. Nurses were our gate keepers and reviewed all new ideas. They identified and invited patients to participate in the activities while they remained ready to intervene if patients suddenly became critically symptomatic. Each week, I met with the artists and guided their introduction to the nursing units. The nurse director managed the logistics, creating a safe environment where the artists were free to create their art. Importantly, this interprofessional team opened the doors to the clinical areas where artists worked at the bedside with patients and families for the first time ever.

When the beautiful dancer arrived, she walked into the first patient's room. She moved like an angel, floating with colorful scarves twirling around the room; the child opened his eyes in awe, and there was magic. They danced in a new reality of beauty, of connection, of caring through art. The artist painted and created mosaics; the musician played the harp and sang; the poet created poems with patients. The storyteller sat and told stories with families in the waiting rooms. The playback theater group created a clown troupe. Everyone arrived from all over the country. We seized the day! Caring, loving, healing; it was happening.

## ARTS AS ADVANCED NURSING INTERVENTIONS

The integration of the arts into health care was actually advanced nursing intervention therapeutics, described by Dr. Watson as "advanced practice." The artistic activities could, in fact, become part of patient care. Dr. Watson described the arts as healing and caring modalities, encouraging me to bring the arts into the health care system. These arts included painting, music, poetry, dance, meditation, and guided imageries. The theory provided the foundation to expand nursing practice and integrate the arts as nursing as modalities to offer at the bedside.

Nurses were the facilitators for the artists who coexisted in their sacred space. Nurses provided leadership and clinical expertise, emerging as the liaisons with the artists and their allies to bring arts into the hospital space. The theory provided a vision, the framework to orchestrate the artists in healing through their art. The artists entered patients' rooms as they were receiving their chemotherapy or engaged in other treatments. The artists played music, danced, drew, and sculpted. The patients could watch and listen or ask the artist to do what they wanted them to do; the patients could engage in creating art with the artist. It began as one artist in the bone marrow transplant unit (where the average length of stay was 6 weeks) and grew until there were 23 at a time, and then 250 artists. As the program gained statewide recognition, we were asked to help others start similar programs. There are at least five other programs in the state that began with our handbook and training for Shands Hospital's Arts in Medicine.

Staff converted an office space into an art studio for the art supplies, music boxes, music, guided imagery tapes, and the art carts. Nurses initiated patient referrals and invited artists into their patients' rooms. The relationship between artists and patients was part of the therapeutic nursing relationship and the clinical care provided by nursing. In reality, an art session was a caring moment, an encounter between the nursing staff, artist, and the patient/family. It was majestic. When we began this program, about 50% of our patients died in the course of bone marrow transplantation. The Arts in Medicine program honored the expression of both positive and negative feelings (Caritas Process #5; Watson, 2008) that patients/families face amidst the challenges of difficult side effects of therapy and/or end-of-life care.

So what happened? The art encounter created a sacred space for caring–healing at the deepest level. The intention was to make art in whatever way it was expressed. There was no agenda, just an openness to be present and authentic in the moment. It provided the patient with an opportunity for honesty, for engagement, or not. It was based on the readiness of the patient, and each artist/nurse approached the patient without pressure to make art. Sometimes it was simply a time to sit together in silence or to sing a song. It was revealed to be an act of loving-kindness, to be present, to be open, to trust and have faith in the person's abilities and choices. There was a focus on honoring the individual's spiritual expression of faith and desires. For example, the Healing Wall project was created by patients with thousands of tiles that expressed the multiple faiths in the community. The art allows the freedom of expression, of faith, of hope, and of creativity.

The program thrives because it is grounded in this caring–healing arts reality. Theory is a way "to see" (Watson, 2008), to know, and to understand. Caring Science allowed me to see what was happening, to know the truth, and to empower nurses. Since this remarkable project, UF Health nursing chose Caring Science as their nursing theory. Caring Science dwells in the hearts of nurses. It is already what we know to be our practice. The theory merely reminds us of what we are, of what we do, and of who we are.

Nurses are the leaders and the caregivers in the hospital setting. They are constantly at the bedside as all the care is offered in the energetic field of nursing practice. The nurses are the environment of caring. The nurses create the unitary field of consciousness, which resides within each patient encounter and is embraced and embodied in caring consciousness. It is about compassion. The integration of the arts into the institutional darkness of hospitals, with the isolation, fear, illness, science, outcome markers, and now the business-driven system, brings in the light.

## DR. JEAN WATSON—HIGH PRIESTESS OF THE DIVINE FEMININE

How did this theory change my life? It has become my daily spiritual ritual that I practice with my whole being. It is my intention to be more caring, more compassionate, and more loving. It is not easy. My nature is strong. I want to dance to my own music, to be outspoken, and to be defiant. When I discovered art as my way to healing, I had an inspiration to bring it into health care. I had a vision of bringing artists into the hospital rooms to invite everyone to make art. Everyone is an artist and a healer of themselves! In 1990, when I flew to Denver to study Jean's work, my life, my work, my whole being changed. It was a gradual process of living and becoming, being, and knowing. I have grown in so many ways.

Memories are precious. In the remote beautiful country of Bhutan, I was on a pilgrimage with Jean Watson and a few companions. It was a trek up the mountain to visit a sacred monastery, Tiger's Nest, which was built on the side of a cliff. It was going back in time; we carried prayer flags and lit our candles. The younger monks carried bundles of wood up every day. It was a holy place.

We found the inner chamber when the first monk had meditated and become an eternal body of light. I crawled into the small room, found a place among the others, sat down, and prayed. I experienced a moment of total enlightenment; I found the deepest peace I had ever known. I never wanted to leave. It was eternal bliss. Soon, I felt a small tap telling me it was time to go. I took a deep breath. I had discovered a place inside so deep, so vast, and so peaceful. I turned to go; I paused at the door looking out over the incredible beautiful valley. This was not my place to live; I had to go home. I was so happy, the happiest I ever felt. I became so excited that I started to run down the mountain, playing with my companions to chase them down. As I was running down the mountain, I tripped over a rock and fell down. Jean reached out her hand to catch me. She said, "Mary, be careful. Be full of grace and care." I took her hand. She led me the way back home into the light of caring, peace, and my life. The wind twirled around both of us; this is what I heard.

> You are the Light. Listen to the return of the Oracle. The Voice of the Divine Muse; she dances, she sings, she plays, she makes art, she gives birth, she takes death. She is the radiance of the Divine. She is an Oracle that was lost thousands of years ago. Her voice has returned from the depths of lost memories. Her voice speaks to us once again. We can remember what we always knew to be true but had forgotten. She speaks to us today. Listen. She speaks. She teaches us about caring. . . .

Dr. Jean Watson is a Distinguished Professor Emerita, Founder of the Watson Caring Science Institute, and High Priestess of the Divine Feminine.

## ■ REFERENCES

Benson, H. (1975). *The relaxation response.* New York, NY: William Morrow.

Rockwood Lane, M. (2010). *Mary's story.* Retrieved from www.maryrockwoodlane.com

Siegel, B. (2011). *About Bernie Siegel.* Retrieved from www.berniesiegelmd.com

University of Massachusetts Medical School. (2014). *Faculty biography: John Kabat-Zinn.* Retrieved from http://www.umassmed.edu/cfm/about-us/people/2-meet-our-faculty/kabat-zinn-profile

Watson, J. (1999). *Postmodern nursing and beyond.* London, England: Churchill Livingstone.

Watson, J. (2002). Intentionality and caring-healing consciousness: A practice of transpersonal nursing. *Holistic Nursing Practice, 16*(4), 12–19.

Watson, J. (2008). *Nursing: The philosophy and science of caring.* Boulder, CO: University Press of Colorado.

Watson, J. (2012). *Human caring science: A theory of nursing* (2nd ed.). Sudbury, MA: Jones & Bartlett.

# Index

authentic presence, Watson's, 27
authentically present, as key element, 189–190

biogenic environments, 146

Canadian Institutes of Health Research (CIHR), 127
CARE. *See* Collaborative Action Research and Evaluation
caring–healing accomplishments
    arts in medicine, 222–223
    divine feminine, 224–225
    nursing interventions, 223–224
*The Caring Imperative in Education* (Watson), 34
caring leadership, 67
    professional practices, 67–68
caring ontology
    nursing research method, 104
    operationalization of, 106–107
Caring Patient Assessment Scale (CPAS), 147–150
Caring Science, 29–31
    key elements, 60, 133–135
Caring Science, Mindful Practice, 26, 29–31
Caring Science and care
    CARE, 119–120
    participatory paradigm, 120–121
    perspectives, 49–50
    relational ontology, 121–122
    shared values, shared foundations, 117–119
Caring Science and Caritas, 26
    being-in-relation, 134–135
    implementation of theory, 135–136
    intentionality, 135
    journey, 4–5, 14, 24–26, 34, 60, 90–91, 102–103, 132–133, 164–165, 188–189, 218
    key elements, 157–161, 165–166
    literacy, 116, 156–157

praying research, 138–139
    Ukraine, 136–138
Caring Science Theory, 35
caring theory-infused practices, 93–94
Caritas Coach Education Program (CCEP), 63
Caritas Illiteracy, 7
Caritas Literacy
    authentic presence, 62–63
    geriatric caring model, 19
    health systems, 19
    key elements, 60
    knowing/being/doing/becoming, 36–40
    mindful-awareness, 60–61
    persons with dementia, 17–18
    primary palliative, 18–19
    reflective practice, 60–61
    self-care, 62
    vulnerability, 61–62
Caritas-informed practice
    new space for, 84
CCEP. *See* Caritas Coach Education Program
CIHR. *See* Canadian Institutes of Health Research
Collaborative Action Research and Evaluation (CARE), 116
community-based research (CBR)
    methodology, 126
    methods, 126–127
conscious awareness, 27
CPAS. *See* Caring Patient Assessment Scale
creating heart-centered leadership, 96–97
Critical Caritas Literacy, 6–7
    creating discourse and practices for, 8
    discourse and practices for, 8
    ontological practices, 7
    unfinished ontological guides, 9–10
critical literacy, 5–6
    Watson's guide, 8
cultural exchange in research approach, 145
cybercaring text, 31

digital world, 26
divine order, 220–221

education in research approach, 145
environment, healing, 28
ethical demand, 38
Europe
    Bologna agreements, 45–46
    French-speaking world, 44–45
    history and pedagogical evolution, 44
    La Source, 46–47
    nursing science in, 44
evolution in research approach, 145
expert support in research approach, 145
extended epistemology
    axiology, 125–126
    empirical (or propositional) knowing, 123
    experiential knowing, 122
    practical knowing, 123–124
    praxis, 124–125
    presentational knowing, 123

fostering heart-centered leadership, 91–93

global nursing knowledge development, 73–74

healing, Caritas arts for, 218–225
healing environment, 28
healing with arts, 221

individual studies in research approach, 145
International Hiroshima Caring and Peace
    Conference–March 2012, 211–212

Japanese Caritas
    Caring Science leadership, 211
    continuing Caritas, 213
    peace and change, 210–211
Japanese Red Cross College of Nursing–Tokyo
    Research Program, 213–215

leadership
    caring leadership, 67–68
    disciplinary perspective on, 67

global research and scholarship, 65–67
journey, 63
love and caring, 26–27
loving-kindness, 221

massive open online course (MOOC), 29–31
Middle East nurses
    caring practices, practical applications of,
        206–207
    health, understandings of, 203–205
    language, 202
    multicultural care, 200–202
    religion and tradition, 202–203
    stereotypes, 205–206
midwifery
    caring moment, 165–166
    Caring Science and Caritas, 165
    Caritas processes, 166–167
    conceptual framework for, 167–168
    South Africa, 168–170
    Watson's theory in, 170
mindful practice text, 29–31
MOOC. *See* massive open online course

Nhat Hahn, Thich, 27
nurse faculty leader, 65
nursing research method
    caring ontology, 104
    caring theory, 105
    relevance of creating, 103–104
    research participants, 105
*Nursing: The Philosophy and Science of*
    *Caring*, 8

paternalistic sociomedical culture, 75–76
Peru
    communitas, 85–86
    context for change, 76–77
    global nursing knowledge, 73–74
    nurse-led project exemplar, 81–83
    paternalistic sociomedical culture, 75–76
    political action, 84
    situational assessment, 76
    South America, transitioning caring to,
        74–75
    space and building, 79–80
    translating caring to achieve outcomes, 79
practice in research approach, 145